# Current Concepts in the Management of Pathologic Conditions

*Editor*

JOHN H. CAMPBELL

# ORAL AND MAXILLOFACIAL SURGERY CLINICS OF NORTH AMERICA

www.oralmaxsurgery.theclinics.com

*Consulting Editor*
RICHARD H. HAUG

February 2013 • Volume 25 • Number 1

**ELSEVIER**

1600 John F. Kennedy Boulevard • Suite 1800 • Philadelphia, Pennsylvania, 19103-2899

www.theclinics.com

ORAL AND MAXILLOFACIAL SURGERY CLINICS OF NORTH AMERICA Volume 25, Number 1
February 2013 ISSN 1042-3699, ISBN-13: 978-1-4557-7129-5

Editor: John Vassallo; j.vassallo@elsevier.com
Developmental Editor: Teia Stone

*Oral and Maxillofacial Surgery Clinics of North America* (ISSN 1042-3699) is published quarterly by Elsevier Inc., 360 Park Avenue South, New York, NY 10010-1710. Months of issue are February, May, August, and November. Business and Editorial Offices: 1600 John F. Kennedy Blvd., Suite 1800, Philadelphia, PA 19103-2899. Periodicals postage paid at New York, NY and additional mailing offices. Subscription prices are $369.00 per year for US individuals, $543.00 per year for US institutions, $165.00 per year for US students and residents, $431.00 per year for Canadian individuals, $645.00 per year for Canadian institutions, $495.00 per year for international individuals, $645.00 per year for international institutions and $224.00 per year for Canadian and foreign students/residents. To receive student/resident rate, orders must be accompanied by name or affiliated institution, date of term, and the *signature* of program/residency coordinator on institution letterhead. Orders will be billed at individual rate until proof of status is received. Foreign air speed delivery is included in all *Clinics* subscription prices. All prices are subject to change without notice. **POSTMASTER:** Send address changes to *Oral and Maxillofacial Surgery Clinics of North America,* Elsevier Periodicals Customer Service, 11830 Westline Industrial Drive, St. Louis, MO 63146. Tel: 1-800-654-2452 (U.S. and Canada); 314-447-8871 (outside U.S. and Canada). Fax: 314-447-8029. E-mail: journalscustomerservice-usa@elsevier.com (for print support); journalsonlinesupport-usa@elsevier.com (for online support).

*Reprints.* For copies of 100 or more, of articles in this publication, please contact the Commercial Reprints Department, Elsevier Inc., 360 Park Avenue South, New York, NY 10010-1710. Tel.: 212-633-3812; Fax: 212-462-1935; Email: reprints@elsevier.com.

*Oral and Maxillofacial Surgery Clinics of North America* is covered in *MEDLINE/PubMed (Index Medicus)*, *Science Citation Index Expanded (SciSearch®)*, *Journal Citation Reports/Science Edition*, and *Current Contents®/Clinical Medicine*.

Printed and bound by CPI Group (UK) Ltd, Croydon, CR0 4YY

Transferred to digital print 2012

# Contributors

## CONSULTING EDITOR

**RICHARD H. HAUG, DDS**
Carolinas Center for Oral Health,
Charlotte, North Carolina

## EDITOR

**JOHN H. CAMPBELL, DDS, MS**
Associate Professor and Residency Director,
Department of Oral and Maxillofacial Surgery,
School of Dental Medicine, University at
Buffalo; Staff Surgeon, Erie County Medical
Center, Buffalo, New York

## AUTHORS

**JUSTIN AU, DMD, MD**
Chief Resident, Department of Oral and
Maxillofacial Surgery, University at Buffalo,
Buffalo, New York

**R. BRYAN BELL, DDS, MD, FACS**
Head and Neck Surgical Associates; Affiliate
Professor of Oral and Maxillofacial Surgery,
Oregon Health and Science University; Medical
Director, Oral, Head and Neck Cancer
Program, Robert W. Franz Cancer Research
Center, Providence Cancer Center; Attending
Surgeon, Legacy Emanuel Medical Center,
Portland, Oregon

**TUAN G. BUI, MD, DMD**
Attending Surgeon, Head and Neck Surgical
Associates, Legacy Emanuel Medical Center
and Providence Portland Cancer Center;
Affiliate Assistant Professor of Oral and
Maxillofacial Surgery, Oregon Health and
Science University, Portland, Oregon

**JOHN H. CAMPBELL, DDS, MS**
Associate Professor and Residency Director,
Department of Oral and Maxillofacial Surgery,
School of Dental Medicine, University at
Buffalo; Staff Surgeon, Erie County Medical
Center, Buffalo, New York

**ERIC R. CARLSON, DMD, MD, FACS**
Professor and Kelly L. Krahwinkel
Chair, Department of Oral and Maxillofacial
Surgery; Director, Oral and Maxillofacial
Surgery Residency Program; Director of
Oral/Head and Neck Oncologic Surgery
Fellowship Program, University of
Tennessee Graduate School of Medicine;
Chief, Head and Neck Service, University
of Tennessee Cancer Institute, Knoxville,
Tennessee

**HEIDI C. CROW, DMD, MS**
Associate Professor, Department of Oral
Diagnostic Sciences, University at Buffalo,
Buffalo, New York

**ERIC J. DIERKS, DMD, MD, FACS**
Director of Fellowship in Head and Neck
Oncologic and Microvascular Reconstructive
Surgery, Head and Neck Surgical Associates,
Legacy Emanuel Medical Center and
Providence Portland Cancer Center; Affiliate
Professor of Oral and Maxillofacial Surgery,
Oregon Health and Science University,
Portland, Oregon

**G.E. GHALI, DDS, MD, FACS**
Gamble Professor and Chairman, Department of Oral and Maxillofacial/Head and Neck Surgery, Louisiana State University Health Science Center Shreveport, Shreveport, Louisiana

**YOLY GONZALEZ, DDS, MS, MPH**
Assistant Professor, Department of Oral Diagnostic Sciences, University at Buffalo, Buffalo, New York

**JOSEPH I. HELMAN, DMD**
Chalmers J. Lyons Endowed Professor and Chair, Department of Oral and Maxillofacial Surgery, Taubman Center, University of Michigan, Ann Arbor, Michigan

**D. DAVID KIM, DMD, MD, FACS**
Associate Professor, Department of Oral and Maxillofacial/Head and Neck Surgery, Louisiana State University Health Science Center Shreveport, Shreveport, Louisiana

**ETERN S. PARK, DDS, MD**
Fellow in Head and Neck Oncologic Surgery, Head and Neck Surgical Associates, Legacy Emanuel Medical Center and Providence Portland Cancer Center, Portland, Oregon

**DHAVAL PATEL, DDS**
Resident, Department of Oral and Maxillofacial Surgery, University at Buffalo, Buffalo, New York

**M.A. POGREL, DDS, MD, FRCS, FACS**
Professor and Chair, Department of Oral and Maxillofacial Surgery, University of California San Francisco, San Francisco, California

**SALVATORE L. RUGGIERO, DMD, MD, FACS**
New York Center for Orthognathic and Maxillofacial Surgery, Lake Success; Clinical Professor, Department of Oral and Maxillofacial Surgery, School of Dental Medicine, SUNY at Stony Brook, New York; Clinical Professor, Hofstra LIJ-North Shore School of Medicine, Hempstead, New York

**JAMES J. SCIUBBA, DMD, PhD**
Formerly, Professor, Departments of Otolaryngology-Head and Neck Surgery, Pathology, and Dermatology, Johns Hopkins School of Medicine, Baltimore; Presently, Consultant at the Milton J. Dance Head and Neck Cancer Center, Greater Baltimore Medical Center, Baltimore, Maryland

**JONATHAN W. SHUM, DDS, MD**
Fellow in Microvascular Reconstructive Surgery, Head and Neck Surgical Associates, Legacy Emanuel Medical Center and Providence Portland Cancer Center, Portland, Oregon

**BRENT B. WARD, DDS, MD**
Associate Professor and Fellowship Program Director, Oral and Maxillofacial Surgery, Maxillofacial Oncologic and Reconstructive Surgery, University of Michigan, Ann Arbor, Michigan

**DAVID E. WEBB, MAJ, USAF, DC**
Staff Oral and Maxillofacial Surgeon, David Grant Medical Center, Travis Air Force Base, California

**MELVYN S. YEOH, DMD, MD**
Assistant Professor, Department of Oral and Maxillofacial/Head and Neck Surgery, Louisiana State University Health Science Center Shreveport, Shreveport, Louisiana

# Contents

Several studies have reported the prevalence of pathology associated with retained third molar teeth. Although most oral surgeons have encountered many patients with infection and lytic lesions associated with retained third molars, assessment of the frequency of abnormality around these teeth has previously been hampered by the lack of well-designed studies to investigate a subject so important to oral and maxillofacial surgeons. This article reviews what is known—and what isn't known—about pathologic conditions associated with both symptomatic and asymptomatic third molar teeth.

Since the first description of bone necrosis in patients receiving bisphosphonate therapy in 2004, there have been multiple retrospective, prospective, and case-control studies that have served to characterize the diagnosis, associated risk factors, and treatment of this new complication. Bisphosphonate-related osteonecrosis of the jaw is at present associated with several risk factors that are identified across several disciplines in medicine and dentistry. With this level of broad-based recognition, new clinical and basic science research initiatives have begun and are likely to elucidate the etiopathogenesis of this disease process, significantly improving the level of disease management and prevention.

In 2005, the World Health Organization renamed the lesion previously known as an odontogenic keratocyst as the keratocystic odontogenic tumor. The clinical features associated with the keratocystic odontogenic tumor show it to be a unilocular or multilocular radiolucency, occurring most frequently in the posterior mandible. These tumors are normally diagnosed histologically from a sample of the lining. With simple enucleation, it seems that the recurrence rate may be from 25% to 60%.

A specific and regimented approach to the diagnosis and management of patients with disease of the parotid gland is necessary for correct diagnosis and management. Patient morbidity or mortality may result if there is a delay in the diagnosis of a malignant parotid tumor. This article reviews the diagnosis and management of parotid disease, with a particular concentration on neoplastic processes. An overview of the superficial parotid mass is emphasized because most neoplastic processes occupy the superficial lobe of the parotid gland.

medical oncologists. In recent years, great scientific progress has been made in targeted therapies. Although many modalities remain in preclinical validation, some advances affect patient care today. This article summarizes the concepts of targeting and explores current examples of successful targeting and emerging targeting technologies in head and neck oncology.

Oral lichen planus is a common immunologically mediated mucocutaneous disease. These lesions have varied clinical presentations and symptoms, which include reticular, erosive, or erythematous forms. This article reviews the diagnosis and management of oral lichen planus.

# ORAL AND MAXILLOFACIAL SURGERY CLINICS OF NORTH AMERICA

**THE CLINICS ARE NOW AVAILABLE ONLINE!**
Access your subscription at:
**www.theclinics.com**

# Preface
# Current Concepts in the Management of Pathologic Conditions

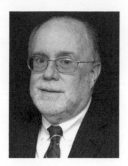

John H. Campbell, DDS, MS
*Editor*

Just a couple of days ago, as I was making dinner for the family (self-preservation in my household), my 17-year-old daughter strolled into the kitchen.

*"Something's wrong with my gum behind the last tooth—it's swollen and it hurts!"*

Her complaint, heard hundreds of times per day in oral surgery practice, highlights the need for definitive guidance in our approach to management of the third molar. Should *all* third molars be removed? Only the symptomatic ones? And what is third molar pathology anyway?

Fortunately, increasing numbers of well-designed studies have provided insight into areas of pathologic abnormality encountered by each of us on a regular basis. This issue was conceived to highlight advances in knowledge, review difficult-to-manage conditions, and introduce the reader to new technologies that will impact the health of our patients, now and in the future.

Some of the articles published here discuss conditions commonly seen in daily practice; others present current understanding of less regularly encountered disease, and a few shine light on innovations so new that they are—at present—available in only a few teaching centers. Each will provide information valuable to surgical practice, and I encourage you to read every one of them. You won't be disappointed.

As guest editor, I extend my appreciation to each of the authors represented in this volume. It is no small effort to research, organize, write, and rewrite a review article, sometimes sifting through hundreds of books and periodicals to cull the truth from an overabundance of published information. I think you, the reader, will find their endeavors worthwhile.

As always, a few acknowledgments are in order. I am grateful for the assistance of Elsevier editor John Vassallo; his regular reminders encouraged all of us to complete assignments—if not in a timely fashion, at least in the proper fashion (and I understand his stress ulcers are better now). Edward Leisner, librarian at the Erie County Medical Center, was most helpful in acquiring necessary articles. Jason Chwirut, assistant media specialist at the University at Buffalo, ably assisted with illustrations.

And my daughter? Her mother (my supervisor both at the University and at home) is a dentist. She was pleased to refer me to the guidelines on third molars published by the National Institute for Clinical Excellence: third-molar extraction isn't indicated until the *second* episode of pericoronitis. I sure hope that doesn't happen on prom night...

John H. Campbell, DDS, MS
University at Buffalo
School of Dental Medicine
112 Squire Hall
3435 Main Street
Buffalo, NY 14214, USA

E-mail address:
jc294@buffalo.edu

http://dx.doi.org/10.1016/j.coms.2012.11.009
1042-3699/13/$ – see front matter © 2013 Published by Elsevier Inc.

oralmaxsurgery.theclinics.com

# Pathology Associated with the Third Molar

John H. Campbell, DDS, MS

## KEYWORDS

- Third molar • Wisdom tooth • Pathology • Cyst

## KEY POINTS

- Erupted, disease-free third molar teeth may be retained indefinitely.
- Periodontal abnormality is common at third molar sites, and may be difficult to control or eradicate with conventional periodontal therapy techniques because of abnormal eruption patterns or proximity of teeth to the mandibular ramus.
- Third molar sites commonly harbor microbial flora known to be associated with periodontal disease, and evidence suggests that third molar sites may first be affected by periodontitis that moves to more anterior locations over time.
- The periodontal status of second molars tends to improve after extraction of third molars that exhibit periodontal abnormality.
- Pericoronal tissue that is histologically indistinguishable from a dentigerous cyst may affect greater than one-third of impacted third molars without abnormal pericoronal radiolucency, and this is more common in patients after age 20 years.
- At present, the relationship of retained third molars to systemic disease is tenuous.

## INTRODUCTION

There has been much discussion in the literature regarding the prevalence of third molar pathology and extraction.[1–6] The cost to the individual and to society (in the form of lost productivity), and the morbidity associated with surgery for third molar extraction, seems to form the basis for many investigators to discourage extraction of asymptomatic teeth. So-called prophylactic extraction of third molar teeth has, in fact, been deemed a "public health hazard."[7] Lack of symptoms has led investigators to recommend retention of third molars[8]; others recommend a watchful waiting approach, and intervention when disease is identified.[4,5] Few published articles, however, have taken into account the possibility of early or occult disease that could be eliminated by intervention before symptom development, and it has

been rightly recognized that lack of symptoms does not necessarily equate to lack of disease.[2] Just as no dentist would fail to treat a carious lesion because it is asymptomatic, the surgeon should recognize that the presence (and sometimes likelihood) of asymptomatic disease may necessitate extraction of retained third molars at an age when morbidity is likely to be less and recovery faster.

As it has been recognized that third molars that are not fully erupted commonly change position over time (even past the "normal" eruption age), it is prudent to monitor retained teeth for development of pathosis for a lifetime.[9–12] For example, in one 5-year study where retained third molar teeth were monitored, it was necessary to extract about one-third of them during the time frame of the investigation,[13] and it is still unclear as to whether the majority of third molar teeth can be retained in a reasonable state of health as individuals age.

Department of Oral and Maxillofacial Surgery, School of Dental Medicine, University at Buffalo, 3435 Main Street, #112 Squire Hall, Buffalo, NY 14214, USA
E-mail address: jc294@buffalo.edu

Oral Maxillofacial Surg Clin N Am 25 (2013) 1–10
http://dx.doi.org/10.1016/j.coms.2012.11.005
1042-3699/13/$ – see front matter © 2013 Elsevier Inc. All rights reserved.

Disease associated with third molar teeth may be clinically obvious or occult. Although tooth pain is commonly associated with third molars,[14] patients will frequently present with nebulous complaints of headache, "pressure," or pain that is not readily attributable to the teeth. In many of these scenarios, clinical examination will not be able to definitively attribute the symptoms to the third molars. The surgeon is then faced with the dilemma of recommending retention or extraction for a given individual. It is hoped that the following discussion will aid in both the diagnosis and management of these patients.

For the purposes of this article, pathologic manifestations will be divided into soft-tissue conditions (primarily pericoronitis and periodontal disease), conditions affecting hard tissues of teeth, and lytic lesions of bone. Each is discussed in turn.

## SOFT-TISSUE CONDITIONS
### Pericoronitis and Infection

Pericoronitis, an inflammatory condition associated with the soft tissue around a partially erupted third molar, commonly occurs when a lower third molar tooth cannot erupt fully and remains partially covered by a soft-tissue operculum because of its position in the jaw (**Fig. 1**). It has been suggested that the teeth most likely to develop pericoronitis are vertically positioned lower third molars at or near the level of the occlusal plane,[15–18] but pericoronitis is also seen in a high percentage of orthodontically treated cases with mesioangular position of the lower third molars.[19] In some cases, pericoronitis may be chronic and painless[20] with only intermittent symptoms, but is often acutely recurrent in a specific individual. The gingival tissues may be exquisitely tender and purulent, causing significant discomfort for the patient,

and limiting jaw opening and chewing function. In certain circumstances, as with deployed service personnel, the condition can be particularly problematic.[21] There is also evidence that mandibular third molar pericoronitis may be associated with more underlying periodontal inflammatory disease in young adults when compared with a similar population without pericoronitis,[22] and, even 3 months after removal of offending teeth, microbial loads and inflammatory mediators may remain elevated.[16]

Ample peer-reviewed literature has reported the flora associated with both acute and chronic pericoronitis.[23–28] Many of the bacterial species are facultative or obligate anaerobes, and several species have been identified as periodontal pathogens.[25,29,30] Some data, however, suggest that the flora is more consistent with gingivitis than periodontitis.[16] Older published literature may not provide a complete picture of the bacterial flora associated with this condition because it is based on culture techniques that are not capable of growing all microbial species present. Newer molecular methodologies have discovered several uncultivable organisms not previously identified at third molar sites, and it has been suggested by some investigators that the soft tissues around third molars with acute or chronic pericoronitis may provide a niche for the establishment of periodontal abnormality at other oral sites.[29]

Pericoronitis may be managed with a variety of interventions, including subgingival curettage to remove plaque and foreign bodies, irrigation with antimicrobials such as chlorhexidine, or antibiotic therapy. Operculectomy, although sometimes effective in reducing symptoms in the short term, does not appear to provide long-term benefit for most patients.[31] In cases where the erupted or partially erupted upper third molar impinges on a lower operculum, extraction of the upper third molar may aid pain control and speed the healing process. Extraction of the lower third molar tooth is generally indicated for patients once any infection and swelling have resolved, especially if recurrent.[32]

Although most cases of pericoronitis will resolve with local intervention, a small percentage will progress to major infection. The frequency of this outcome is reported to be low, however: on the order of 0.016 cases per year per 1000 patients at risk.[33] Such individuals are seriously ill, often demonstrating multispace infections compromising the airway, and requiring intubation, extensive drainage procedures in the operating room, and critical-care management for several days. It appears that most hospitalizations result from diseased third molars or nonelective removal of

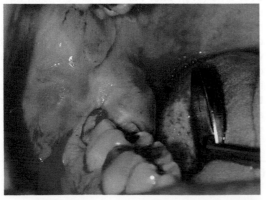

**Fig. 1.** Third molar demonstrating pericoronitis with operculum and associated swelling.

diseased third molars.[34,35] Fortunately, death is rare.

Acute or chronic symptoms thought to be related to third molars have also been reported to delay the diagnosis and treatment of cancer in a small number of cases.[36] Clinicians should, of course, be aware that pain or other symptoms at third molar sites may reflect more serious conditions than localized pericoronitis.

## Periodontal Disease

There is mounting evidence that asymptomatic third molar teeth, especially lower third molar teeth, are frequently associated with pathologic periodontal probing depths.[37] In addition, the gingivae around these teeth have been repeatedly shown to harbor bacteria known to be associated with the development of periodontitis. Some investigators have demonstrated that these pathogenic bacteria are found first at third molar sites, which may thus serve as a reservoir for the development of more generalized periodontal disease.[29,38] In addition, there is evidence that removal of third molars reduces the presence of periodontopathic bacteria at second molar sites.[39] These findings suggest that early removal of lower third molars unlikely to erupt into a healthy periodontal state may prevent or delay the onset of adult periodontitis. In addition, they suggest that periodontal probing should be an integral part of clinical assessment to adequately advise the patient about retention or extraction of third molars.

As already indicated, periodontal pathogens are commonly found in pericoronal tissues of third molar teeth, and have been reported even in otherwise periodontally healthy individuals.[25] Periodontal pocketing and increased inflammatory mediators may be found even in patients with asymptomatic third molars.[40] Not surprisingly, periodontal abnormality at third molar sites increases over time in young adults,[3,41] and is seen more frequently in third molars than in first or second molars in this population.[42] It has also been suggested that chronic oral inflammation leads to progression of periodontal disease in the third molar region,[43] and that the presence of visible third molars may negatively affect periodontal health.[44] Visible third molars, however, have also been associated with periodontal inflammatory disease in non–third molar sites in young adults[45]; this is more likely for mandibular third molars than for maxillary,[46] and periodontal abnormality at third molar sites is predictive of the same at non–third molar regions over time in the young adult population.[47] In this same population,

periodontal abnormality worsens over time in non–third molar sites, but this is more likely to happen in patients with at least one probing depth of at least 4 mm in the third molar region.[48] These probing depths also indicate a risk for progression of periodontal disease during pregnancy,[49] and have been associated with an increased risk of preterm birth.[50] In a large study of middle-aged and older Americans, fewer than 2% of subjects had third molars free of dental caries or periodontal abnormality,[51] and the presence of a visible third molar was significantly associated with more severe periodontal disease at sites more anterior, particularly on second and first molars.[52] Third molars may continue to negatively affect the health of the periodontium as individuals age.[53]

Improvement in the periodontal status of the second molar over time has been demonstrated after removal of both the lower and upper third molar, at least in younger adults,[54–58] and flap design for extraction does not appear to negatively affect periodontal healing.[59] Improvement in alveolar bone height has been demonstrated at the distal of the second molar after extraction of impacted mandibular third molars in comparison with their retention.[60] In general, second molar periodontal health improves or remains constant after extraction of the third molar. A possible exception to this outcome, however, is the patient with normal periodontal health preoperatively, as these individuals may see the periodontal status of the second molar worsen after third molar extraction[61]; increasing age may also be associated with worsening periodontal status.[62]

## HARD-TISSUE CONDITIONS
## Dental Caries

Certainly the most common hard-tissue disorder associated with third molar teeth is dental caries. Ahmad and colleagues[63] demonstrated that 27% of subjects with caries-free erupting third molars will develop dental caries within 5 years, and Venta and colleagues[64] report a 30% rate of caries or filled surfaces for erupting third molars within 6 years; the prevalence of third molar caries also appears to increase over time.[3] Because many of these teeth are malposed and/or never achieve complete eruption, they may be difficult candidates for dental restoration (**Fig. 2**). In such cases, extraction may be the most efficacious treatment.

In addition to dental caries in the third molar, third molar angulation may predispose to caries on the distal surface of the second molar tooth, with prevalence of second molar caries up to 12.6% in one studied population.[65] Early carious lesions on the second molar can be difficult to

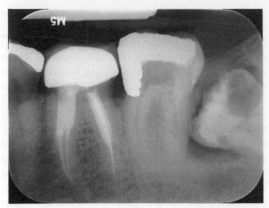

**Fig. 2.** Impacted, symptomatic third molar in a 70-year-old man demonstrating dental caries, lack of bone on the second molar, and pericoronal radiolucency.

distinguish from so-called cervical burnout, and treatment may thus not occur in the early stages of disease. Second molar lesions often begin in the area of the cementoenamel junction because of a mesioangularly or horizontally impacted third molar, and may involve significant portions of the distal second molar root. Resorption of the second molar root may occur even in the absence of dental caries (**Fig. 3**). In advanced lesions, restoration of the second molar is not possible, and both the second and third molar teeth must be extracted.

### Odontogenic Cysts and Tumors

Every oral and maxillofacial surgeon is familiar with displaced third molar teeth associated with large radiolucencies (**Figs. 4–8**). Sometimes associated with pain, swelling, or functional disturbances, these lesions most often have no signs or symptoms, and the condition is discovered incidentally during a radiographic survey. Lesions may occur in any age group, with extremes of

age posing the greatest challenge in management. Because these patients are generally referred to the oral surgeon for diagnosis and management, the population seen by surgeons is skewed toward individuals with disease; what seems common in specialty practice could, in fact, be relatively rare in the general population. The frequency of these lytic lesions thus cannot be determined solely from practice populations because of selection bias in specialty practice. How, then, can the likelihood of cyst or tumor development associated with retained third molar teeth be determined?

The preponderance of literature regarding the development of odontogenic cysts and tumors associated with third molar teeth is radiographic, retrospective, and/or cross-sectional in nature.[66,67] Commonly an author will retrieve existing panoramic radiographs from a series of patients and assess them for the presence of radiolucencies around third molar teeth. Although this provides some information, there are several factors that preclude the ability to assess prevalence of cystic (or tumorous) change. First, many of the radiographs will demonstrate that the third molars are absent because they have previously been removed. Of course, it is not clear if such teeth had been removed to treat disease or if they were extracted prophylactically. Second, a radiographic study of this type cannot rule out early hard-tissue or soft-tissue disease. Panoramic radiography may not demonstrate early dental caries, and developing cysts or tumors may not yet have caused discernible bone destruction. Nevertheless, at least one retrospective study has reported an alarming frequency of radiographically detectable pathosis in 46.4% in 2432 impacted lower third molars,[68] and postorthodontic follow-up radiographs also report pathosis in both third molars and adjacent second molars.[11]

Histologic assessment of tissues remains the gold standard for disease diagnosis, and several

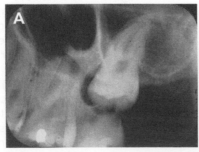

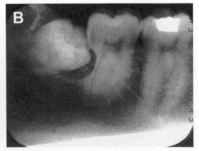

**Fig. 3.** (*A*) Severe second molar root resorption caused by maxillary third molar. (*B*) Severe second molar root resorption caused by mandibular third molar (same patient as in *A*). This individual had similar findings on all second molars.

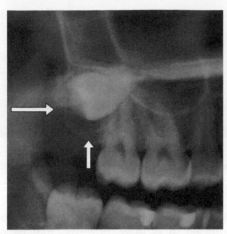

**Fig. 4.** Arrows illustrate typical small dentigerous cyst surrounding a maxillary third molar tooth in a female patient.

peer-reviewed publications have reported findings when soft tissues associated with third molars were analyzed histologically.[69,70] Some of these report retrospectively only on findings from submitted tissues (ie, only when the surgeon deemed the tissues obviously pathologic),[71,72] and frequency of reported pathologic change varies widely, less than 10% in some reports.[73] Others report some disease entity in nearly 60% of pericoronal tissues of unerupted third molars[74]: chronic soft-tissue inflammation and dentigerous cysts were commonly encountered; odontogenic tumors or malignancies were rare. Manganaro[75] demonstrated similar findings, with a dentigerous cyst reported in nearly 46% of pericoronal radiolucencies (0.1–3.0 mm) around impacted third molar teeth. Several recent studies have evaluated soft tissues retrieved from third molar sites without radiographic evidence of disease (follicular spaces 3 mm or less), and have reported pathologic change in high percentages, greater than 50% in some reports.[76,77] Inflammatory changes and

cyst formation are common in pericoronal tissues of even fully impacted asymptomatic third molars.[78]

Glosser and Campbell[79] designed a prospective evaluation of soft tissues from third molars without radiographic evidence of disease (less than 2.5 mm pericoronal radiolucency). Tissues were evaluated independently by 3 different oral pathologists, and only when all 3 agreed that a specimen represented disease was the tissue deemed to be pathologic. In this study, 31 of 96 specimens were diagnosed as dentigerous cyst; no other pathologic lesions were identified.

A similar trend was reported by Adelsperger and colleagues,[80] in whose study 99 specimens were evaluated independently by 2 oral pathologists. In the event of a disagreement in diagnosis, a consensus diagnosis was achieved. Surprisingly, 34% of the specimens were found to represent dentigerous cysts, concurring nearly exactly with the findings reported by Glosser. In this study, however, a subset of follicular and cystic tissues was further assessed for the presence of proliferating cell nuclear antigen (PCNA), a marker of active cellular division. A high percentage of positivity was found in the cystic tissues (62.5%), whereas none of the examined follicular tissues showed mitotic activity. Although there were no gender differences in the percentage of cystic tissues, the actively growing cysts were associated with increasing age, suggesting that these may have become radiographically evident at some future time. Others have also associated a higher frequency of cystic change in patients older than 20 years,[70,74] and Daley and Wysocki[81] reported that approximately 30% of dentigerous cysts in a large pathology database occurred in patients older than 39 years.

A third histologic analysis attempted to correlate patient symptoms with the presence of cysts.[82] Patients presenting to a private oral surgeon completed a questionnaire regarding their perceptions

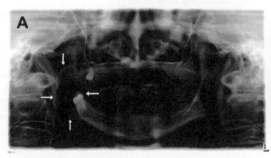

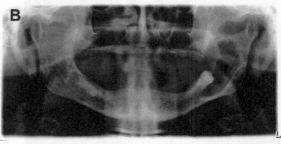

**Fig. 5.** (*A*) Dentigerous cyst associated with a displaced, impacted third molar tooth in a 94-year-old woman (*white arrows*). Red arrow indicates impacted maxillary third molar with discontinuity in overlying bone but no overt disease. (*B*) Similar dentigerous cyst in an 83-year-old male patient.

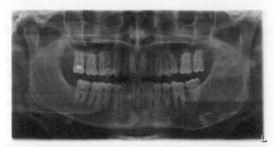

**Fig. 6.** Cemento-ossifying fibroma associated with a displaced third molar tooth in a 21-year-old man.

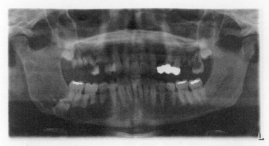

**Fig. 8.** Odontogenic keratocyst in association with a displaced third molar in a 59-year-old male patient.

of symptoms associated with their third molar teeth. Again, pericoronal tissues were submitted for histologic diagnosis, and again nearly one-third of sites were found to have dentigerous cysts. On analysis, however, symptoms of infection, swelling, pain, or "pressure" showed no correlation with the location of the cysts. Nearly equal percentages of cysts and follicles had some symptom, and symptoms could thus not predict which teeth harbored odontogenic cysts.

Some controversy exists among pathologists regarding the diagnosis of dentigerous cysts. Whereas many consider squamous metaplasia of pericoronal tissues to indicate the diagnosis, others argue that histology alone cannot confirm the presence of cystic change.[81,83–86] The findings of increased cellular activity demonstrated by some of the previously referenced investigators support the conclusion that the histologic findings represent pathosis. Whether these actively growing tissues continue to grow, become

quiescent, or involute over time has yet to be determined. It is likely, however, that because pericoronal tissues are not routinely submitted for histologic diagnosis, associated disease is underdiagnosed.

## SUMMARY

Controversy continues to cloud the issue of third molar retention, although enough information is available for the surgeon to make informed decisions in recommending retention or extraction for his or her patients. The following points should be considered when advising patients:

- Erupted, disease-free third molar teeth may be retained indefinitely
- "Asymptomatic" does not mean "disease-free"
- Periodontal abnormality is common at third molar sites, and may be difficult to control or eradicate with conventional periodontal therapy techniques because of abnormal eruption patterns or proximity of teeth to the mandibular ramus
- Third molar sites commonly harbor a microbial flora known to be associated with periodontal disease, and evidence suggests that third molar sites may first be affected by periodontitis that moves to more anterior locations over time
- Acute or chronic pericoronitis sites may also harbor periodontal pathogens
- The periodontal status of second molars tends to improve after extraction of third molars that exhibit periodontal abnormality
- Pericoronal tissue that is histologically indistinguishable from dentigerous cyst may affect greater than one-third of impacted third molars without abnormal pericoronal radiolucency, and this is more common in patients after age 20 years
- Symptoms do not correlate with the location of most dentigerous cysts

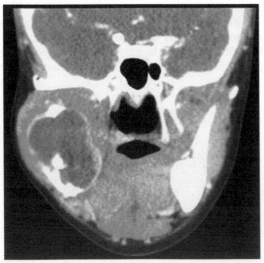

**Fig. 7.** A displaced third molar associated with ameloblastic carcinoma in an 11-year-old male patient.

- Third molar position may change long after the "normal" eruption time
- At present, the relationship of retained third molars to systemic disease is tenuous

The surgeon would do well to incorporate periodontal probing into the examination of the third molar for documentation of periodontal abnormality associated with erupted, partially erupted, and impacted third molar teeth. Patients who elect to retain third molars should undergo clinical and radiographic examination regularly (perhaps as frequently as every 2 years) for early diagnosis of disease, because the prevalence of third molar abnormality (especially asymptomatic) appears to be much higher than previously thought. Younger patients unable or unwilling to have regular surveillance may wish to consider removal of teeth at high risk of present or future disease at an age when surgical morbidity is likely to be less.

## REFERENCES

1. Obiechina AE, Arotiba JT, Fasola AO. Third molar impaction: evaluation of the symptoms and pattern of impaction of mandibular third molar teeth in Nigerians. Odontostomatol Trop 2001;24:22–5.
2. White RP Jr, Proffit WR. Evaluation and management of asymptomatic third molars: lack of symptoms does not equate to lack of pathology. Am J Orthod Dentofacial Orthop 2011;140:10–7.
3. Fisher EL, Garaas R, Blakey GH, et al. Changes over time in the prevalence of caries experience or periodontal pathology on third molars in young adults. J Oral Maxillofac Surg 2012;70:1016–22.
4. Hill CM. Removal of asymptomatic third molars: an opposing view. J Oral Maxillofac Surg 2006;64: 1816–20.
5. Kandasamy S. Evaluation and management of asymptomatic third molars: watchful monitoring is a low-risk alternative to extraction. Am J Orthod Dentofacial Orthop 2011;140:10–7.
6. Kandasamy S, Rinchuse DJ. The wisdom behind third molar extractions. Aust Dent J 2009;54:284–92.
7. Friedman JW. The prophylactic extraction of third molars: a public health hazard. Am J Public Health 2007;97:1554–9.
8. Sasano T, Kuribara N, Iikubo M, et al. Influence of angular position and degree of impaction of third molars on development of symptoms: long-term follow-up under good oral hygiene conditions. Tohoku J Exp Med 2003;200:75–83.
9. Phillips C, Norman J, Jaskolka M, et al. Changes over time in position and periodontal probing status of retained third molars. J Oral Maxillofac Surg 2007; 65:2011–7.
10. Venta I, Turtola L, Ylipaavalmiemi P. Radiographic follow-up of impacted third molars from age 20 to 32 years. Int J Oral Maxillofac Surg 2001;30:54–7.
11. Kahl B, Gerlach KL, Hilgers RD. A long-term, follow-up, radiographic evaluation of asymptomatic impacted third molars in orthodontically treated patients. Int J Oral Maxillofac Surg 1994;23:279–85.
12. Sewerin I, von Wowern N. A radiographic four-year follow-up study of asymptomatic mandibular third molars in young adults. Int Dent J 1990;40:24–30.
13. Hill CM, Walker RV. Conservative, non-surgical management of patients presenting with impacted lower third molars: a 5-year study. Br J Oral Maxillofac Surg 2006;44:347–50.
14. Samsudin AR, Mason DA. Symptoms from impacted wisdom teeth. Br J Oral Maxillofac Surg 1994;32: 380–3.
15. Hazza'a AM, Bataineh AB, Odat AA. Angulation of mandibular third molars as a predictive factor for pericoronitis. J Contemp Dent Pract 2009;10:51–8.
16. Blakey GH, White RP Jr, Offenbacher S, et al. Clinical/biological outcomes of treatment for pericoronitis. J Oral Maxillofac Surg 1996;54:1150–60.
17. Halverson BA, Anderson WH 3rd. The mandibular third molar position as a predictive criteria for risk for pericoronitis: a retrospective study. Mil Med 1992;157:142–5.
18. Leone SA, Edenfield MJ, Cohen ME. Correlation of acute pericoronitis and the position of the mandibular third molar. Oral Surg Oral Med Oral Pathol 1986;62:245–50.
19. Gungormus M. Pathologic status and changes in mandibular third molar position during orthodontic treatment. J Contemp Dent Pract 2002;3:11–22.
20. Laine M, Venta I, Hyrkas T, et al. Chronic inflammation around painless partially erupted third molars. Oral Surg Oral Med Oral Pathol Oral Radiol Endod 2003;95:277–82.
21. Combes J, McColl E, Cross B, et al. Third molar related morbidity in deployed service personnel. Br Dent J 2010;209:E6.
22. Gelesko S, Blakey GH, Partrick M, et al. Comparison of periodontal inflammatory disease in young adults with and without pericoronitis involving mandibular third molars. J Oral Maxillofac Surg 2009;67:134–9.
23. Sixou JL, Migaud C, Jolilvet-Gougeon A, et al. Evaluation of the mandibular third molar pericoronitis flora and its susceptibility to different antibiotics prescribed in France. J Clin Microbiol 2003;41: 5794–7.
24. Sixou JL, Magaud C, Jolivet-Gougeon A, et al. Microbiology of mandibular third molar pericoronitis: incidence of beta-lactamase-producing bacteria. Oral Surg Oral Med Oral Pathol Oral Radiol Endod 2003;95:655–9.
25. Rajasuo A, Sihvonen OJ, Peltola M, et al. Periodontal pathogens in erupting third molars of periodontally

healthy subjects. Int J Oral Maxillofac Surg 2007;36: 818–21.

26. Leung WK, Theilade E, Comfort MB, et al. Microbiology of the pericoronal pouch in mandibular third molar pericoronitis. Oral Microbiol Immunol 1993;8: 306–12.

27. Mombelli A, Buser D, Lang NP, et al. Suspected periodontopathogens in erupting third molar sites of periodontally healthy individuals. J Clin Periodontol 1990;17:48–54.

28. Hurlen B, Olsen I. A scanning electron microscopic study on the microflora of chronic periocoronitis of lower third molars. Oral Surg Oral Med Oral Pathol 1984;58:522–32.

29. Mansfield JM, Campbell JH, Bhandari AR, et al. Molecular analysis of 16S rRNA genes identifies potentially pathogenic bacteria and archaea in the plaque of partially erupted third molars. J Oral Maxillofac Surg 2012;70:1507–14.

30. Peltroche-Llacsahuanga H, Reichart E, Schmitt W, et al. Investigation of infectious organisms causing pericoronitis of the mandibular third molar. J Oral Maxillofac Surg 2000;58:611–6.

31. Ness GM, Peterson LJ. Impacted teeth. In: Miloro M, editor. Peterson's principles of oral and maxillofacial surgery, vol. 1, 2nd edition. Hamilton (New Zealand): BC Decker; 2004. p. 141.

32. National Institute for Clinical Excellence. Guidance on the extraction of wisdom teeth. 2000. Available at: www.nice.org.uk/nicemedia/pdf/wisdomteethguidance. pdf. Accessed November 6, 2012.

33. Berge TI. Incidence of infections requiring hospitalization associated with partially erupted third molars. Acta Odontol Scand 1996;54:309–13.

34. Kunkel M, Morbach T, Kleis W, et al. Third molar complications requiring hospitalization. Oral Surg Oral Med Oral Pathol Oral Radiol Endod 2006;102: 300–6.

35. Kunkel M, Kleis W, Morbach T, et al. Severe third molar complications including death—lessons from 100 cases requiring hospitalization. J Oral Maxillofac Surg 2007;65:1700–6.

36. Venta I, Oikarinen VJ, Soderholm AL, et al. Third molars confusing the diagnosis of carcinoma. Oral Surg Oral Med Oral Pathol 1993;75:551–5.

37. Blakey GH, Marciani RD, Haug RH, et al. Periodontal pathology associated with asymptomatic third molars. J Oral Maxillofac Surg 2002;60:1227–33.

38. White RP Jr, Madianos PN, Offenbacher S, et al. Microbial complexes detected in the second/third molar region in patients with asymptomatic third molars. J Oral Maxillofac Surg 2002;60:1234–40.

39. Rajasuo A, Meurman JH, Murtomaa H. Periodontopathic bacteria and salivary microbes before and after extraction of partly erupted third molars. Scand J Dent Res 1993;101:87–91.

40. White RP Jr, Offenbacher S, Phillips C, et al. Inflammatory mediators and periodontitis in patients with asymptomatic third molars. J Oral Maxillofac Surg 2002;60:1241–5.

41. Blakey GH, Jacks MT, Offenbacher S, et al. Progression of periodontal disease in the second/third molar region in subjects with asymptomatic third molars. J Oral Maxillofac Surg 2006;64:189–93.

42. Garass RN, Fisher EL, Wilson GH, et al. Prevalence of third molars with caries experience or periodontal pathology in young adults. J Oral Maxillofac Surg 2012;70:507–13.

43. White RP Jr, Offenbacher S, Blakey GH, et al. Chronic oral inflammation and the progression of periodontal pathology in the third molar region. J Oral Maxillofac Surg 2006;64:880–5.

44. Elter JR, Cuomo CJ, Offenbacher S, et al. Third molars associated with periodontal pathology in the Third National Health and Nutrition Examination Survey. J Oral Maxillofac Surg 2004;62: 440–5.

45. Blakey GH, Gelesko S, Marciani RD, et al. Third molars and periodontal pathology in American adolescents and young adults: a prevalence study. J Oral Maxillofac Surg 2010;68:325–9.

46. Blakey GH, Golden BA, White RP Jr, et al. Changes over time in the periodontal status of young adults with no third molar periodontal pathology at enrollment. J Oral Maxillofac Surg 2009;67:2425–30.

47. White RP Jr, Phillips C, Hull DJ, et al. Risk markers for periodontal pathology over time in the third molar and non-third molar regions in young adults. J Oral Maxillofac Surg 2008;66:749–54.

48. Blakey GH, Hull DJ, Haug RH, et al. Changes in third molar and nonthird molar periodontal pathology over time. J Oral Maxillofac Surg 2007;65:1577–83.

49. Moss KL, Ruvo AT, Offenbacher S, et al. Third molars and progression of periodontal pathology during pregnancy. J Oral Maxillofac Surg 2007;65: 1065–9.

50. Moss KL, Mauriello S, Ruvo AT, et al. Reliability of third molar probing measures and the systemic impact of third molar periodontal pathology. J Oral Maxillofac Surg 2006;64:652–8.

51. Garass R, Moss KL, Fisher EL, et al. Prevalence of visible third molars with caries experience or periodontal pathology in middle-aged and older Americans. J Oral Maxillofac Surg 2011;69: 463–70.

52. Moss KL, Oh ES, Fisher E, et al. Third molars and periodontal pathologic findings in middle-age and older Americans. J Oral Maxillofac Surg 2009;67: 2592–8.

53. Elter JR, Offenbacher S, White RP, et al. Third molars associated with periodontal pathology in older Americans. J Oral Maxillofac Surg 2005;63:179–84.

54. Montero J, Mazzaglia G. Effect of removing an impacted mandibular third molar on the periodontal status of the mandibular second molar. J Oral Maxillofac Surg 2011;69:2691–7.

55. Coleman M, McCormick A, Laskin DM. The incidence of periodontal defects distal to the maxillary second molar after impacted third molar extraction. J Oral Maxillofac Surg 2011;69:319–21.

56. Dicus C, Blakey GH, Faulk-Eggleston J, et al. Second molar periodontal inflammatory disease after third molar removal in young adults. J Oral Maxillofac Surg 2010;68:3000–6.

57. Blakey GH, Parker DW, Hull DJ, et al. Impact of removal of asymptomatic third molars on periodontal pathology. J Oral Maxillofac Surg 2009; 67:245–50.

58. Faria AI, Gallas-Torreira M, Lopez-Raton M. Mandibular second molar periodontal healing after impacted third molar extraction in young adults. J Oral Maxillofac Surg 2012;70:2732–41.

59. Chaves AJ, Nascimento LR, Costa ME, et al. Effects of surgical removal of mandibular third molar on the periodontium of the second molar. Int J Dent Hyg 2008;6:123–8.

60. Krausz AA, Machtei EE, Peled M. Effects of lower third molar extraction on attachment level and alveolar bone height of the adjacent second molar. Int J Oral Maxillofac Surg 2005;34:756–60.

61. Dodson TB, Richardson DT. Risk of periodontal defects after third molar surgery: an exercise in evidence-based clinical decision-making. Oral Maxillofac Surg Clin North Am 2007;19:93–8.

62. Kugelberg CF. Impacted lower third molars and periodontal health. An epidemiological, methodological, retrospective and prospective clinical, study. Swed Dent J Suppl 1990;68:1–52.

63. Ahmad N, Gelesko S, Shugars D, et al. Caries experience and periodontal pathology in erupting third molars. J Oral Maxillofac Surg 2008;66:948–53.

64. Venta I, Meurman JH, Murtomaa H, et al. Effect of erupting third molars on dental caries and gingival health in Finnish students. Caries Res 1993;27: 438–43.

65. Polat HB, Ozan F, Kara I, et al. Prevalence of commonly found pathoses associated with mandibular impacted third molars based on panoramic radiographs in Turkish population. Oral Surg Oral Med Oral Pathol Oral Radiol Endod 2008;105: e41–7.

66. Stanley HR, Alattar M, Collett WK, et al. Pathological sequelae of "neglected" impacted third molars. J Oral Pathol 1988;17:113–7.

67. Alattar M, Baughman RA, Collett WA. A survey of panoramic radiographs for evaluation of normal and pathologic findings. Oral Surg Oral Med Oral Pathol 1980;50:472–8.

68. Al-Khateeb TH, Bataineh AB. Pathology associated with impacted mandibular third molars in a group of Jordanians. J Oral Maxillofac Surg 2006;64: 1598–602.

69. Yildirim G, Ataoglu H, Mihmanli A, et al. Pathologic changes in soft tissues associated with asymptomatic impacted third molars. Oral Surg Oral Med Oral Pathol Oral Radiol Endod 2008;106:14–8.

70. Baykul T, Baglam AA, Aydin U, et al. Incidence of cystic changes in radiographically normal impacted lower third molar follicles. Oral Surg Oral Med Oral Pathol Oral Radiol Endod 2005;99:542–5.

71. Stathopoulos P, Mezitis M, Kappatos C, et al. Cysts and tumors associated with impacted third molars: is prophylactic removal justified? J Oral Maxillofac Surg 2011;69:405–8.

72. Guven O, Keskin A, Akal UK. The incidence of cysts and tumors around impacted third molars. Int J Oral Maxillofac Surg 2000;29:131–5.

73. Brkic A, Mutlu S, Kocak-Berberoglu H, et al. Pathological changes and immunoexpression of p63 gene in dental follicles of asymptomatic impacted lower third molars. J Craniofac Surg 2010;21: 854–7.

74. Raprasitkul S. Pathologic change in the pericoronal tissues of unerupted third molars. Quintessence Int 2001;32:633–8.

75. Manganaro AM. The likelihood of finding occult histopathology in routine third molar extractions. Gen Dent 1998;46:200–2.

76. Mesgarzadeh AH, Esmailzadeh H, Abdolrahimi M, et al. Pathosis associated with radiographically normal follicular tissues in third molar impactions. Indian J Dent Res 2008;19:208–12.

77. Kotrashetti VS, Kale AD, Bhalaerao SS, et al. Histopathologic changes in soft tissue associated with radiographically normal impacted third molars. Indian J Dent Res 2010;21:385–90.

78. Simsek-Kaya G, Ozbek E, Kalkan Y, et al. Soft tissue pathosis associated with asymptomatic impacted lower third molars. Med Oral Patol Oral Cir Bucal 2011;16:e929–36.

79. Glosser JW, Campbell JH. Pathologic change in soft tissues associated with radiographically "normal" third molar impactions. Br J Oral Maxillofac Surg 1999;37:259–60.

80. Adelsperger J, Campbell JH, Coates DB, et al. Early soft tissue pathosis associated with impacted third molars without pericoronal radiolucency. Oral Surg Oral Med Oral Pathol Oral Radiol Endod 2000;89: 402–6.

81. Daley TD, Wysocki GP. The small dentigerous cyst: a diagnostic dilemma. Oral Surg Oral Med Oral Pathol Oral Radiol Endod 1995;79:77–81.

82. Campbell JH, Coates DB, Summerlin D-J, et al. Are third molar symptoms associated with the presence

of dentigerous cysts? J Oral Maxillofac Surg 2005; 63(Suppl 1):38.

83. Kim J, Ellis GL. Dental follicular tissue: misinterpretation as odontogenic tumors. J Oral Maxillofac Surg 1993;51:762–7.

84. Eisenberg E. Discussion: dental follicular tissue: misinterpretation as odontogenic tumors. J Oral Maxillofac Surg 1993;51:767–8.

85. Damante JH, Fleury RN. A contribution to the diagnosis of the small dentigerous cyst or the paradental cyst. Pesqui Odontol Bras 2001;15: 238–46.

86. Stanley HR, Krogh H, Pannkuk E. Age changes in the epithelial components of follicles (dental sacs) associated with impacted third molars. Oral Surg Oral Med Oral Pathol 1965;19:128–39.

# Emerging Concepts in the Management and Treatment of Osteonecrosis of the Jaw

Salvatore L. Ruggiero, DMD, MD[a,b,c,*]

## KEYWORDS

- Osteonecrosis • BRONJ • Jaw necrosis • Bisphosphonates • Bone remodeling
- Antiresorptive treatment

## KEY POINTS

- Bisphosphonate-related osteonecrosis of the jaw is now a well-recognized entity that is associated with several risk factors that are identified across several disciplines in medicine and dentistry.
- Although osteonecrosis of the jaw (ONJ) has been well described in the literature, the pathogenesis of this disease process remains poorly understood.
- Standardization of diagnostic criteria and nomenclature for this clinical entity is important to facilitate future clinical and epidemiologic research.
- The goal of treatment of patients at risk of developing ONJ, or for those who have active disease, is preservation of quality of life by controlling pain, managing infection, and preventing the development of new areas of necrosis.

Since the first description of bone necrosis in patients receiving bisphosphonate therapy in 2004, there have been multiple retrospective, prospective, and case-control studies that have served to characterize the diagnosis, associated risk factors, and treatment of this new complication. Although bisphosphonate-related ONJ was not well recognized 10 years ago, it is at present associated with several risk factors that are identified across several disciplines in medicine and dentistry. With this level of broad-based recognition, new clinical and basic science research initiatives have begun and are likely to elucidate the etiopathogenesis of this disease process, significantly improving the level of disease management and prevention.

## PATHOGENESIS

Despite the fact that ONJ has been well described in the literature, the pathogenesis of this disease process remains poorly understood. Four major hypotheses have been proposed to explain the etiology of the disease process, including bone remodeling suppression (osteoclast mediated), disturbances in bone vascularity (antiangiogenesis), local mucosal toxicity, and genetic factors.

The most popular and researched hypothesis focuses on the profound inhibition of osteoclast function associated with these drugs. Bisphosphonate-mediated suppression of bone remodeling is thought to have a greater effect in the jaw, where baseline bone turnover rates are typically much higher than at other skeletal sites.

Disclosure: Consultant for Amgen Inc.

[a] New York Center for Orthognathic and Maxillofacial Surgery, 2001 Marcus Avenue, Suite N10, Lake Success, NY 11042, USA; [b] Department of Oral and Maxillofacial Surgery, School of Dental Medicine, SUNY at Stony Brook, Stony Brook, South Drive, NY 11794, USA; [c] Department of Dental Medicine, Hofstra LIJ-North Shore School of Medicine, Hofstra Northern Boulevard, Hempstead, NY 11549, USA

* New York Center for Orthognathic and Maxillofacial Surgery, 2001 Marcus Avenue, Suite N10, Lake Success, NY 11042.

E-mail address: drruggiero@nycoms.com

Oral Maxillofacial Surg Clin N Am 25 (2013) 11–20
http://dx.doi.org/10.1016/j.coms.2012.10.002
1042-3699/13/$ – see front matter © 2013 Elsevier Inc. All rights reserved.

This position is supported by several studies that have demonstrated bone necrosis isolated to the alveolar component of the jaw in animal models exposed to bisphosphonates.[1–3]

The finding that nonbisphosphonate osteoclast inhibitors may be associated with osteonecrosis also supports this hypothesis. Denosumab (Prolia, Xgeva) is a novel antiresorptive agent and a fully humanized antibody against RANKL. It is a profound inhibitor of osteoclast function and bone remodeling. These agents do not bind to bone, and their affects on bone remodeling are reversible within 6 months of treatment cessation. Recent case reports,[4–6] as well as reports from large-scale clinical trials,[7] have shown that ONJ occurs in patients treated with denosumab. These findings strongly suggest that potent remodeling suppression in the form of osteoclast inhibition, a common feature of both denosumab and the bisphosphonates, is likely a key factor in the pathogenesis of ONJ (**Fig. 1**).

Defects of angiogenesis have also been considered as a mechanism for ONJ. This idea has been fueled by reports of bisphosphonate-induced inhibition of angiogenesis in culture and animal tumor models.[8,9] These findings, however, are tempered by other animal studies in which bisphosphonates had no effect on angiogenesis associated with endochondral ossification[10] and findings of normal vasculature in regions of bisphosphonate-induced matrix necrosis.[1]

Direct mucosal toxicity from high bisphosphonate concentrations in the bone has been considered as the primary event for jawbone exposure and necrosis.[11] This idea is based on culture data in which high concentrations of bisphosphonates were found to be toxic to oral mucosal cells. In the clinical setting, such an effect would occur only if the oral mucosa were subject to high concentrations of bisphosphonate for a prolonged period. This situation can theoretically occur at surgical sites or regions of inflammation where there is a local reduction in the pH, which facilitates the release of bisphosphonate from the bone.[12] The clinical scenario where ONJ presents spontaneously in the nondentate region of the jaw, however, does not fit this hypothesis well.

The fact that only a small subset of patients exposed to bisphosphonates develop jaw necrosis has led some investigators to consider certain pharmacogenetic factors as well.[13,14] In particular, Sarasquette[15] noted certain genetic irregularities (ie, single nucleotide polymorphisms) in the cytochrome P450-2C gene in patients with multiple myeloma and ONJ. Patients who were homozygous for the T allele had a 12.7-fold increased risk of developing ONJ. The link to ONJ formation is thought to be related to alterations in bone vascularity and arachidonic acid metabolism, both of which are controlled by this gene.

All these studies provide a much greater understanding of this disease process and certainly provide a clearer direction to which future research should be directed. The degree to which any of these theories, working in concert or individually, can completely explain the development of this drug-mediated bone necrosis remains to be determined more fully. Considering the aforementioned studies, ONJ can be accurately predicted based on specific risk factors such as the presence of jaw inflammation (trauma or infection), a genetic marker, and antiresorptive bone therapy.

## CLINICAL PRESENTATION AND DIAGNOSIS

Standardization of diagnostic criteria and nomenclature for this clinical entity is important to facilitate future clinical and epidemiologic research. In addition, a uniform definition for ONJ serves to distinguish this new clinical entity from other delayed intraoral healing conditions. Various organizations have proposed clinical definitions for ONJ, all of which are analogous to each other; this has resulted in some degree of confusion. This condition has been referred to in the literature by several acronyms, including BRONJ (bisphosphonate-related osteonecrosis of the jaw), BRON (bisphosphonate-related osteonecrosis), BON (bisphosphonate osteonecrosis), BAONJ (bisphosphonate associated osteonecrosis of the jaw), and simply ONJ.

The American Association of Oral and Maxillofacial Surgeons (AAOMS) established a working definition for BRONJ, which has remained unchanged since it was first defined in 2006. The tenets of the diagnosis include (1) an exposure

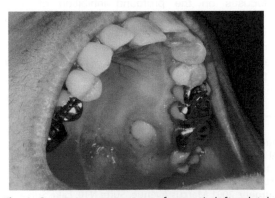

**Fig. 1.** Spontaneous exposure of necrotic left palatal bone (stage 1) in a patient receiving denosumab for the treatment of metastatic lung cancer. The patient had no history of bisphosphonate exposure.

history to bisphosphonates, (2) exposed bone within the oral cavity, and (3) no history of prior radiation therapy to the jaws. The emergence of jaw necrosis in bisphosphonate-naive patients receiving RANKL inhibitors,[4–7] however, may necessitate a modification of these criteria in the near future. The ADA later introduced the more generic term ARAONJ (antiresorptive associated osteonecrosis of the jaw) to include those new cases of necrosis associated with monoclonal therapy. Despite the variations in nomenclature, the clinical finding of exposed, necrotic bone remains the consistent hallmark of the diagnosis, and therefore physical examination is the most effective method of establishing the diagnosis of jaw necrosis.

The differential diagnosis of ONJ should exclude other common clinical conditions including, but not limited to, alveolar osteitis, sinusitis, gingivitis/periodontitis, periapical pathology, and temporomandibular joint disorders. In those rare situations in which exposed bone is present in patients exposed to bisphosphonates and radiation therapy to the jaw, osteoradionecrosis should be strongly considered. Although bone inflammation and infection are typically present in patients with advanced ONJ, this is a secondary event. The exposed bone and surrounding soft tissue become secondarily infected, presenting a clinical scenario that is similar to osteomyelitis. The histologic analysis of these bone specimens, however, rarely demonstrates the criteria required to establish a diagnosis of acute or chronic osteomyelitis. Analyses of the physical properties of the resected necrotic bone have also failed to demonstrate any unique features that would serve as a reliable biomarker for this disease process.[16,17]

The patient history and clinical examination remain the most sensitive diagnostic tools for this condition. Areas of exposed and necrotic bone may remain asymptomatic for weeks, months, or even years. These lesions are most frequently symptomatic when the surrounding tissues become inflamed or there is clinical evidence of exposed bone. Signs and symptoms that may occur before the development of clinically detectable osteonecrosis include pain, tooth mobility, mucosal swelling, erythema, and ulceration. These symptoms may occur spontaneously or, more commonly, at the site of prior dentoalveolar surgery. Most case series have described this complication at regions of previous dental surgery (ie, extraction sites); exposed bone, however, has also been reported in patients with no history of trauma or in edentulous regions of the jaw. Intraoral and extraoral fistulae may develop when necrotic jawbone becomes secondarily infected. Some patients

may also present with complaints of altered sensation in the affected area as the neurovascular bundle becomes compressed from the inflamed surrounding bone. Chronic maxillary sinusitis secondary to osteonecrosis with or without an oral-antral fistula can be the presenting symptom in patients with maxillary bone involvement.

It has been observed that lesions are found more commonly in the mandible than in the maxilla (2:1 ratio). They are also more prevalent in areas with thin mucosa overlying bone prominences such as tori, exostoses, and the mylohyoid ridge.[18–20] The size of the affected area is variable and ranges from a nonhealing extraction site to exposure and necrosis of large sections of jawbone. The area of exposed bone is typically surrounded by inflamed erythematous soft tissue. Purulent discharge at the site of exposed bone is present when these sites become secondarily infected. Microbial cultures from areas of exposed bone usually show normal oral microbes and therefore are not always helpful. In cases in which there is extensive soft-tissue involvement, however, microbial culture data may define comorbid oral infections that may facilitate the selection of an appropriate antibiotic regimen.

A clinical staging system developed by Ruggiero and colleagues[19] and adopted by the AAOMS in 2006[21] and updated in 2009[22] has served to categorize patients with ONJ, direct rational treatment guidelines, and collect data to assess the prognosis and treatment outcome in patients who have used either intravenous (IV) or oral bisphosphonates (Table 1). Patients with no evidence of exposed or necrotic bone are considered to be "at risk" if they have been exposed to either IV or oral bisphosphonates. The potency of the bisphosphonate used, the duration of exposure, and dentoalveolar surgery seem to be the main determinants in assessing the risk of developing ONJ. Patients with stage 1 disease have exposed bone but are asymptomatic. There is no evidence of significant adjacent or regional soft-tissue inflammatory swelling or infection. Patients may have symptoms of pain before the development of radiographic changes suspicious for osteonecrosis or clinical evidence of exposed bone. Stage 2 disease is characterized by exposed bone with associated pain, adjacent or regional soft-tissue inflammatory swelling, or secondary infection. Patients with stage 3 disease have exposed bone associated with pain, adjacent or regional soft-tissue inflammatory swelling, or secondary infection in addition to a pathologic fracture, an extraoral fistula, or radiographic evidence of osteolysis extending to the inferior border of the mandible or sinus floor (Fig. 2).

**Table 1**
**Staging of bisphosphonate-related osteonecrosis of the jaw**

| Stage | Findings |
|---|---|
| At-risk category | No apparent exposed/necrotic bone in patients who have been treated with either oral or IV bisphosphonates |
| Stage 0 | Nonspecific clinical findings and symptoms such as jaw pain or osteosclerosis but no clinical evidence of exposed bone |
| Stage 1 | Exposed/necrotic bone in patients who are asymptomatic and have no evidence of infection |
| Stage 2 | Exposed/necrotic bone associated with infection as evidenced by pain and erythema in the region of the exposed bone with or without purulent drainage |
| Stage 3 | Exposed/necrotic bone in patients with pain, infection, and one or more of the following: pathologic fracture, extraoral fistula, or osteolysis extending to the inferior border or sinus floor |

*Data from* Advisory Task Force on Bisphosphonate-Related Osteonecrosis of the Jaws. American Association of Oral and Maxillofacial Surgeons position paper on bisphosphonate-related osteonecrosis of the jaws. J Oral Maxillofac Surg 2007;65:369.

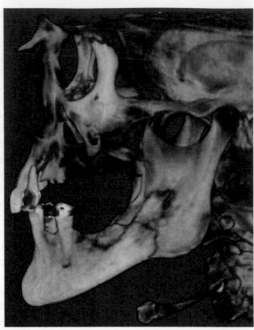

**Fig. 2.** Three-dimensional CT image of a patient with stage 3 ONJ who presented with a large region of sequestrum and a pathologic fracture of the left mandibular angle. The patient had a diagnosis of stage 4 breast cancer and a history of extensive IV bisphosphonate exposure.

Since the publication of the initial treatment guidelines in 2006, reports of nonspecific signs and symptoms such as pain, abscess formation, altered sensory function, or osteosclerosis have emerged in patients with a bisphosphonate exposure history but no clinical evidence of necrosis. In an effort to determine whether or not these findings represent a precursor for clinical disease, the updated AAOMS position paper has included these patients in a new stage 0 category.[22] The degree to which patients with stage 0 disease progress to overt ONJ remains to be determined and represents an important area for future investigation. Recent reports in the European literature have described a variant of ONJ in which there is bone pain with no exposed bone.[23] Greater than 50% of these patients developed exposed bone at these sites within 5 months.

Multiple risk factors including drug-related issues (potency and duration of exposure), local risk factors (dentoalveolar surgery), local anatomy, concomitant oral and systemic disease, demographic factors, and genetic factors have all been considered for this complication. Only 3 risk factors, however, have remained constant throughout most clinical studies. In most ONJ cases reported to date, recent dentoalveolar trauma was the most prevalent and consistent of these risk factors.[18,24–26] The duration of bisphosphonate therapy also seems strongly related to the likelihood of developing necrosis, with longer treatment regimens associated with a greater risk of developing disease.[25,27] In addition, the more potent IV bisphosphonates that are administered on a monthly schedule such as zoledronic acid and pamidronate are significantly more problematic as compared with other preparations.

Efforts to establish risk assessment by measuring fluctuations in bone turnover markers are problematic and remain controversial.[28–32] The rationale for this approach is based on the knowledge that markers for bone remodeling increase within months after withdrawal of oral bisphosphonate medications, thereby suggesting that osteoclastic function and bone remodeling was normalizing.[33,34] These markers, however, are a reflection of total bone turnover throughout the skeleton and are not specific to the maxilla or mandible where it is suspected that the bone turnover rate may be more severely depressed from prolonged bisphosphonate exposure. From a more practical perspective, using bone turnover markers to estimate the level of bone turnover suppression is only meaningful when compared with baseline pretreatment levels, and these are rarely obtained in clinical practice. In addition, using bone resorption marker levels to assess ONJ risk can be misleading for the small cohort of patients who develop osteoporosis despite normal baseline levels of bone resorption markers.

The radiographic features of ONJ are nonspecific. Plain film radiography does not typically demonstrate any abnormality in the early stages of the disease because of the limited degree of decalcification that is present. Findings on plain film imaging, however, such as localized or diffuse osteosclerosis or a thickening of the lamina dura (components of stage 0), may be predictors for future sites of exposed, necrotic bone. Little or no ossification at a previous extraction site may also represent an early radiographic sign. The findings on computed tomography (CT) are also nonspecific, but this modality is significantly more sensitive to changes in bone mineralization and is therefore more likely to demonstrate areas of focal sclerosis, thickened lamina dura, early sequestrum formation, and presence of reactive periosteal bone (**Fig. 3**). The CT images have also proved to be more accurate in delineating the extent of disease, which is helpful for surgical treatment planning.[35,36] The utility of nuclear bone scanning in patients at risk of ONJ has received growing attention after reports of increased tracer uptake in regions of the jaws that subsequently developed necrosis.[37,38] Although nuclear imaging has limited value in patients with existing disease, its usefulness as

a predictive tool in those patients with preclinical disease (stage 0) seems to have some level of potential benefit and therefore requires continued evaluation.

## TREATMENT AND PREVENTION

The management of patients with ONJ remains challenging because surgical and medical interventions may not eradicate this process. The goal of treatment of patients at risk of developing ONJ, or for those who have active disease, is preservation of quality of life by controlling pain, managing infection, and preventing the development of new areas of necrosis. This treatment has to be balanced with the oncologic management of the patient with osteolytic metastases and the risk of pathologic fracture in the patient with osteoporosis.

Patients at risk of developing ONJ benefit from preventive dental care directed at minimizing the likelihood of extraction and optimizing the level of dental health. The time-tested dental care protocols instituted to prevent osteoradionecrosis in irradiated patients with cancer serve as appropriate models for patients at high risk for ONJ.

The treatment approach for patients with stage 1 disease has remained primarily nonsurgical because these patients are not infected or symptomatic. In most patients with stage 1 disease, the exposed bone eventually matures into a defined sequestrum that can easily be removed. Because infection and pain is typical in patients with stage 2 disease, these patients benefit from local and systemic antibiotic therapy. These patients likewise develop sequestra, which in most cases are managed with local debridement. In patients with stage 3 disease, the extensive nature of the necrosis and infection usually dictate early surgical treatment (segmental resection or marginal resection) for control of the infection and pain (**Fig. 4**).

For those few patients who require surgical resection with a continuity defect, the reconstruction has been challenging. Although there have been reports of immediate reconstruction with vascularized bone grafts, most surgeons are hesitant to proceed with such a procedure because of the uncertain viability of the remaining bone.[39] Alternatively, the mandibular defect can be bridged and stabilized with a reconstruction plate (that could include the condylar head if necessary) and soft-tissue flap. The use of bone morphogenic protein within a sponge carrier has been described for immediate reconstruction of continuity defects in patients with ONJ.[40] This method may represent a viable alternative to autogenous bone grafting

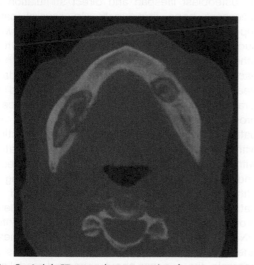

**Fig. 3.** Axial CT scan demonstrating bone sequestration and extensive osteosclerosis in a patient with breast cancer receiving IV bisphosphonate therapy.

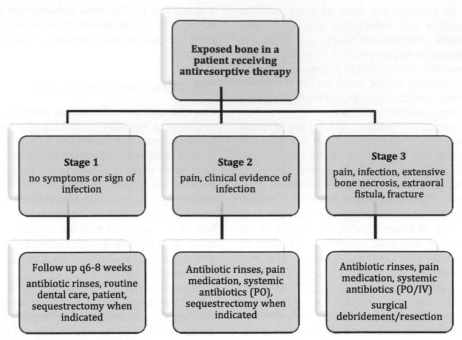

```
                    ┌─────────────────────┐
                    │  Exposed bone in a  │
                    │  patient receiving  │
                    │ antiresorptive therapy│
                    └─────────────────────┘
```

| Stage 1 | Stage 2 | Stage 3 |
|---------|---------|---------|
| no symptoms or sign of infection | pain, clinical evidence of infection | pain, infection, extensive bone necrosis, extraoral fistula, fracture |

| | | |
|---------|---------|---------|
| Follow up q6-8 weeks antibiotic rinses, routine dental care, patient, sequestrectomy when indicated | Antibiotic rinses, pain medication, systemic antibiotics (PO), sequestrectomy when indicated | Antibiotic rinses, pain medication, systemic antibiotics (PO/IV) surgical debridement/resection |

**Fig. 4.** Stage-specific treatment guidelines for ONJ.

techniques in this unique patient population. In the author's experience, immediate reconstruction of maxillectomy defects with an alloplastic obturator has worked well and quickly restored function. Reports from some institutions suggest that early surgical treatment, regardless of disease stage, is associated with a good level of cure and disease control, indicating that surgical treatment may play a larger role in managing this complication in the near future.[39,41–43]

New approaches in the surgical and nonsurgical treatment of ONJ have emerged and may be of value. The use of hyperbaric oxygen (HBO) as an adjunct to nonsurgical therapy has been reported. In a randomized prospective study in which patients received HBO therapy in addition to other forms of care, the treatment group trended better in measurements of pain and quality-of-life score, but healing was only reported in 50% of patients.[44]

The use of platelet-rich plasma as an adjunct to local resection and primary closure was reported in a total of 5 cases at 2 separate institutions.[45,46] In all instances, there was complete wound healing and resolution of pain. However, the small number of cases that were reported and the lack of controls mandate further study before recommending this technique.

In a small case study, simultaneous systemic pentoxifylline (improved microcirculation) and α-tocopherol (antioxidant) administration has been reported to decrease pain and the size of the exposed bone.[47] The rationale for this approach is based on other studies that demonstrated the efficacy of these drugs in the treatment of osteoradionecrosis.

Recombinant human parathyroid hormone (PTH) (teriparatide, Forteo) is the only anabolic agent for bone approved for use in humans in the United States. Daily PTH injections stimulate enhanced bone formation through positive effects on osteoblast lifespan and direct stimulation of quiescent bone lining cells. In several case reports, the use of systemic low-dose PTH was successful in resolving an area of necrosis when other modalities of treatment had failed.[48,49] In each case, when combined with other standard treatment strategies, PTH therapy resulted in a rapid resolution of the exposed bone. In a recent prospective, placebo-controlled study of 40 patients, low-dose systemic PTH in conjunction with vitamin D and oral calcium was associated with greater resolution of periodontal bone defects and accelerated intraoral osseous healing.[50] Although systemic PTH is contraindicated in patients with osteolytic bone metastases, these promising findings may have real applicability for ONJ cases in the noncancer setting. If these agents can be delivered locally to the regions of necrosis, the concern about enhanced medullary cellular proliferation in the patient with cancer may be ameliorated.

## RESEARCH EFFORTS

Since ONJ was first described,[20,51] the importance of developing an adequate animal model to study the factors associated with its cause, presentation, and response to treatment have been realized. Experimental animal models for ONJ have been described within the past several years.[52,53] The challenge for any animal researcher is to establish a model that would be analogous to the human condition in terms of bone healing and response to therapy. It must take into consideration that bone remodeling in humans and large animal species occurs intracortically as opposed to at the bone surface.

In mouse models, bone matrix necrosis and delayed extraction socket healing have been demonstrated in animals exposed to zoledronic acid. Several studies have also focused on the rat model, where exposed bone is noted in a large percentage of extraction sites in animals exposed to bisphosphonates.[54–56] These results are certainly promising and may provide the groundwork for future experiments. A troubling issue for both rodent models, however, is that necrosis also developed in the control groups. The degree to which the findings from these rodent models can be applied to a higher vertebrate biologic system remains to be established. ONJ has also been reported in a dog model, where animals that did not undergo surgery were exposed to various dosages of oral bisphosphonates during a 3-year period. Although there were no areas of exposed bone, large regions of matrix necrosis were identified only within the alveolar bone of the treatment group.[1] Similar results were also seen in dogs treated with oral bisphosphonate for just 1 year.[3] In experiments specifically aimed at understanding the interaction between dental extraction and bisphosphonate exposure in dogs, 1 of 6 animals treated with IV zoledronic acid in doses and schedules comparable to those received by patients with cancer developed exposed, necrotic bone at the extraction sites.[2] These findings in a dog model are encouraging and may develop into a valid animal model for this disease process. Identifying such a model will enable future studies to truly focus on the mechanism of this disease and establish the utility of preventive and management strategies.

## FUTURE CHALLENGES

As one looks at the present understanding of this iatrogenic complication and projects it into the future, there are many questions and challenges that still remain. The emergence of biologic therapies (anti-RANK/RANKL antibodies) as an efficacious bone-targeted treatment of patients with cancer and osteoporosis creates a new set of potential challenges, because these drugs are also associated with the development of jaw necrosis. Although the reversible nature of this humanized antibody may prove to be uniquely beneficial in managing ONJ, those potential benefits have yet to be studied or realized.

Accurate predictors of disease also remain elusive. Although certain types of costly nuclear imaging may prove to have some predictive value for those patients at risk, it remains uncertain as to when or which patients should receive these invasive tests. As yearly zoledronic acid therapy (Reclast) becomes more popular, the ONJ risk assessment needs to be monitored and reassessed. Based on current studies, the risk of developing ONJ was very low through 3 years of yearly zoledronic acid treatment.[57,58] These data need to be considered in comparison to conventional oral bisphosphonate therapy, however, where the risk of developing ONJ usually appears after more than 3 years of exposure. With regard to monthly IV bisphosphonate therapy for cancer, the risk of developing jaw necrosis has been well described, yet the degree and timing (if any) of risk reduction after cessation of therapy remains poorly understood. The variation that exists in the literature regarding how the cumulative dose loads are measured (ie, yes/no, total amount in milligrams, years/months, and total doses) complicates efforts to more precisely assess the exposure risk. This information is pivotal to achieving a better understanding of the exposure thresholds for IV (and oral) therapy so that patients and clinicians are more accurately informed of the progressive risks of these bone-targeted therapies.

The understanding of the etiopathogenesis of this process, although much improved during the past several years, is still lacking. The identification of a reliable animal model system will serve as a valuable experimental tool to assess the various theories of pathogenesis, associated risk factors, and the predictive value of diagnostic and treatment strategies.

## REFERENCES

1. Allen M, Burr D. Mandible matrix necrosis in beagle dogs following 3 years of daily oral bisphosphonate treatment. J Oral Maxillofac Surg 2008;66:987–94.
2. Allen M, Kubek D, Burr D, et al. Compromised osseous healing of dental extraction sites in

zolendronic acid-treated dogs. Osteoporos Int 2010; 22(2):693–702.

3. Burr D, Allen M. Mandibular necrosis in beagle dogs treated with bisphosphonates. Orthod Craniofac Res 2009;12:221–8.

4. Taylor K, Middlefell L, Mizen K. Osteonecrosis of the jaws induced by anti-RANK ligand therapy. Br J Oral Maxillofac Surg 2010;48:221–3.

5. Aghaloo T, Felsenfeld A, Tetradis S. Osteonecrosis of the jaw in a patient on denosumab. J Oral Maxillofac Surg 2010;68:959–63.

6. Diz P, Lopez-Cedrun J, Arenaz J, et al. Denosumab-related osteonecrosis of the jaw. J Am Dent Assoc 2012;143(9):981–4.

7. Stopeck A, Body J, Fujiwara Y. Denosumab versus zolendronic acid for the treatment of breast cancer patients with bone metastases: results of a randomized phase 3 study. Eur J Cancer 2009;7(2): 3082–92.

8. Wood J, Bonjean K, Ruetz S. Novel antiangiogenic effects of the bisphosphonate compound zolendronic acid. J Pharmacol Exp Ther 2002;302: 1055–61.

9. Fournier P, Boissier S, Filleur S, et al. Bisphosphonates inhibit angiogenesis in vitro and testosterone-stimulated vascular regrowth in the ventral prostate in castrated rats. Cancer Res 2002;62:6538–44.

10. Deckers M, Van Beek E, Van Der Pluijm G, et al. Dissociation of angiogenesis and osteoclastogenesis during endochondral bone formation in neonatal mice. J Bone Miner Res 2002;17:998.

11. Landesberg R, Cozin M, Cremers S, et al. Inhibition of oral mucosal cell wound healing by bisphosphonates. J Oral Maxillofac Surg 2008;66:839–47.

12. Otto S, Pautke C, Opelz C, et al. Osteonecrosis of the jaw: effect of BP type, local concentration, and acid milieu on the pathomechanism. J Oral Maxillofac Surg 2010;68:2837–45.

13. Katz J, Gong Y, Salmasinia D, et al. Genetic polymorphisms and other risk factors associated with bisphosphonate induced osteonecrosis of the jaw. Int J Oral Maxillofac Surg 2011;40:605–11.

14. Nicoletti P, Cartsos V, Palaska P, et al. Genomewide pharmocogenetics of bisphosphonate-induced osteonecrosis of the jaw: the role of RBMS3. Int J Oral Maxillofac Surg 2012;17:1–9.

15. Sarasquete M. BRONJ is associated with polymorphisms of the cytochrome P450 CYP2C8 in multiple myeloma: a genome-wide single nucleotide analysis. Blood 2008;111:2709.

16. Allen M, Pandya B, Ruggiero S. Lack of correlation between duration of osteonecrosis of the jaw and sequestra tissue morphology: what it tells us about the condition and what it means for future studies. J Oral Maxillofac Surg 2010;68: 2730–4.

17. Allen M, Ruggiero S. Higher bone matrix density exists in only a subset of patients with bisphosphonate-related osteonecrosis of the jaw. J Oral Maxillofac Surg 2009;67:1373–7.

18. Marx R, Sawatari Y, Fortin M. Bisphosphonate-induced exposed bone (osteonecrosis/osteopetrosis) of the jaws: risk factors, recognition, prevention and treatment. J Oral Maxillofac Surg 2005;63: 1567–75.

19. Ruggiero S, Fantasia J, Carlson E. Bisphosphonate-related osteonecrosis of the jaw: background and guidelines for diagnosis, staging and management. Oral Surg Oral Med Oral Pathol Oral Radiol Endod 2006;102:433–41.

20. Ruggiero S, Mehrotra B, Rosenberg T. Osteonecrosis of the jaws associated with the use of bisphosphonates: a review of 63 cases. J Oral Maxillofac Surg 2004;62:527–34.

21. Advisory Task Force on Bisphosphonate-Related Osteonecrosis of the Jaws, American Association of Oral and Maxillofacial Surgeons. American Association of Oral and Maxillofacial Surgeons. Position paper on bisphosphonate-related osteonecrosis of the jaw. J Oral Maxillofac Surg 2007; 65(3):369–76.

22. Ruggiero S, Dodson T, Assael L, et al. American Association of Oral and Maxillofacial Surgeons position paper on bisphosphonate-related osteonecrosis of the jaws: 2009 update. J Oral Maxillofac Surg 2009;67:2–12.

23. Fedele S, Porter S, D'Aiuto F, et al. Nonexposed variant of bisphosphonate-associated osteonecrosis of the jaw: a case series. Am J Med 2010;123:1060–4.

24. Durie B, Katz M, Crowley J. Osteonecrosis of the jaw and bisphosphonates [letter]. N Engl J Med 2005; 353:99.

25. Badros A, Weikel D, Salama A. Osteonecrosis of the jaw in multiple myeloma patients: clinical features and risk factors. J Clin Oncol 2006;24: 945–52.

26. Barasch A, Cunha-Cruz J, Curro F, et al. Risk factors for osteonecrosis of the jaws: a case-control study from the CONDOR dental PBRN. J Dent Res 2011; 90(4):439–44.

27. Hoff A, Toth B, Altundag K. Osteonecrosis of the jaw in patients receiving intravenous bisphosphonate therapy. J Clin Oncol 2006;24:8528.

28. Bagan J, Jimenez Y, Gomez D, et al. Collagen telopeptide (serum CTX) and its relationship with size and number of lesions in osteonecrosis of the jaws in cancer patients on intravenous bisphosphonates. Oral Oncol 2008;44:1088–9.

29. Kunchur R, Need A, Hughes T, et al. Clinical investigation of C-terminal cross-linking telopeptide test in prevention and management of bisphosphonate-associated osteonecrosis of the jaws. J Oral Maxillofac Surg 2009;67:1167–73.

30. Kwon Y, Kim D, Obe J, et al. Correlation between serum C-terminal cross-linking telopeptide of type 1 collagen and staging of oral bisphosphonate-related osteonecrosis of the jaws. J Oral Maxillofac Surg 2009;67:2644–8.

31. Lehrer S, Montazem A, Ramanathan L, et al. Normal serum bone markers in bisphosphonate-induced osteonecrosis of the jaws. Oral Surg Oral Med Oral Pathol Oral Radiol Endod 2008;106:389–91.

32. Marx R, Cillo J, Ulloa J. Oral bisphosphonate-induced osteonecrosis: risk factors, prediction of risk using serum CTX testing, prevention, and treatment. J Oral Maxillofac Surg 2007;65:2397–410.

33. Rosen H, Moses A, Garber J, et al. Serum CTX: a new marker of bone resorption that shows treatment effect more often than other markers because of low coefficient of variability and large changes with bisphosphonate therapy. Calcif Tissue Int 2000;66:100–3.

34. Rosen H, Moses A, Garber J, et al. Utility of biochemical markers of bone turnover in the follow-up of patients treated with bisphosphonates. Calcif Tissue Int 1998;63:363–8.

35. Treister N, Friedland B, Woo S. Use of cone-beam computerized tomography for evaluation of bisphosphonate-associated osteonecrosis of the jaws. Oral Surg Oral Med Oral Pathol Oral Radiol Endod 2010;109:753–64.

36. Arce K, Assael L, Weissman J, et al. Image findings in bisphosphonate-related osteonecrosis of the jaws. J Oral Maxillofac Surg 2009;67(Suppl 1):75–84.

37. Chiandussi S, Biasotto M, Cavalli F, et al. Clinical and diagnostic imaging of bisphosphonate-associated osteonecrosis of the jaws. Dentomaxillofac Radiol 2006;35:236–43.

38. O'Ryan F, Khoury S, Liao W, et al. Intravenous bisphosphonate-related osteonecrosis of the jaw: bone scintigraphy as an early indicator. J Oral Maxillofac Surg 2009;67:1363–72.

39. Carlson E, Basile J. The role of surgical resection in the mangement of bisphosphonate-related osteonecrosis of the jaws. J Oral Maxillofac Surg 2009; 67(Suppl 1):85–95.

40. Herford A, Boyne P. Reconstruction of mandibular continuity defects with bone morphogenic protein-2 (rhBMP-2). J Oral Maxillofac Surg 2008; 66:616–24.

41. Mucke T, Koschinski J, Deppe H, et al. Outcome of treatment and parameters influencing recurrence in patients with bisphosphonate-related osteonecrosis of the jaws. J Cancer Res Clin Oncol 2011;137(5): 907–13.

42. Stockman P, Vairaktaris E, Wehrhan F, et al. Osteotomy and primary wound closure in bisphosphonate-associated osteonecrosis of the jaw: a prospective clinical study with 12 months follow-up. Support Care Cancer 2009;18:449–60.

43. Stanton DC, Balasanian E. Outcome of surgical management of bisphosphonate-related osteonecrosis of the jaws: review of 33 surgical cases. J Oral Maxillofac Surg 2009;67(5):943–50.

44. Freiberger JJ, Padilla-Burgos R, McGraw T, et al. What is the role of hyperbaric oxygen in the management of bisphosphonate-related osteonecrosis of the jaw: a randomized controlled trial of hyperbaric oxygen as an adjunct to surgery and antibiotics. J Oral Maxillofac Surg 2012;70(7): 1573–83.

45. Curi M, Cossolin G, Koga D, et al. Treatment of avascular necrosis of the mandible in cancer patients with a history of bisphosphonate therapy by combining bone resection and autologous platelet-rich plasma: report of 3 cases. J Oral Maxillofac Surg 2007;65:349–55.

46. Lee C, David T, Nishime M. Use of platelet-rich plasma in the management of oral bisphosphonate-associated osteonecrosis of the jaw: a report of 2 cases. J Oral Implantol 2007;32:371–82.

47. Epstein M, Wicknick F, Eptein J, et al. Management of bisphosphonate-associated osteonecrosis: pentoxifylline and tocopherol in addition to antimicrobial therapy. An initial case series. Oral Surg Oral Med Oral Pathol Oral Radiol Endod 2010;110:593–6.

48. Harper R, Fung E. Resolution of bisphosphonate-associated osteonecrosis of the mandible: possible application for intermittent low-dose parathyroid hormone [rhPTH(1-340]. J Oral Maxillofac Surg 2007;65:573–80.

49. Cheung A, Seeman E. Teriparatide therapy for alendronate-associated osteonecrosis of the jaw. N Engl J Med 2010;363:2473–4.

50. Bashutski JD, Eber RM, Kinney JS, et al. Teriparatide and osseous regeneration in the oral cavity. N Engl J Med 2010;363(25):2396–405.

51. Marx R. Pamidronate (Aredia) and zolendronate (Zometa) induced vascular necrosis of the jaws: a growing epidemic. J Oral Maxillofac Surg 2003; 61:1115–7.

52. Bi Y, Gao Y, Ehirchiou D, et al. Bisphosphonates cause osteonecrosis of the jaw-like disease in mice. Am J Pathol 2010;177:280–90.

53. Kikuiri Y, Kim I, Yamaza T, et al. Cell-based immunotherapy with mesenchymal stem cells cures bisphosphonate-related osteonecrosis of the jaws-like disease in mice. J Bone Miner Res 2010;25: 1668–79.

54. Hokugo A, Christensen R, Chung E, et al. Increased prevalence of bisphosphonate-related osteonecrosis of the jaw with vitamin D deficiency in rats. J Bone Miner Res 2010;25:1337–49.

55. Lopez-Jornet P, Camacho-Alonso F, Molina-Miñano F, et al. An experimental study of bisphosphonate-induced jaw necrosis in Sprague-Dawley rats. J Oral Pathol Med 2010;39(9):697–702.

56. Maahs M, Azambuja AA, Campos MM, et al. Association between bisphosphonates and jaw osteonecrosis: a study in Wistar rats. Head Neck 2011;33(2):199–207.

57. Grbic J, Black D, Lyles K, et al. The incidence of osteonecrosis of the jaw in patients receiving 5 mgs of zolendronic acid. Data from the health outcomes and reduced incidence with zolendronic acid once yearly clinical trials program. J Am Dent Assoc 2010;141:1365–70.

58. Grbic J, Landesberg R, Lin S. Incidence of osteonecrosis of the jaw in women with postmenopausal osteoporosis in the health outcomes and reduced incidence with zolendroic acid once yearly. J Am Dent Assoc 2008;139:32–40.

# The Keratocystic Odontogenic Tumor

M.A. Pogrel, DDS, MD, FRCS

## KEYWORDS

- Keratocystic odontogenic tumor • Odontogenic keratocyst • Enucleation • Radiolucency

## KEY POINTS

- In 2005, the World Health Organization renamed the lesion previously known as an odontogenic keratocyst as the keratocystic odontogenic tumor.
- The clinical features associated with the keratocystic odontogenic tumor show it to be a unilocular or multilocular radiolucency, occurring most frequently in the posterior mandible.
- These tumors are normally diagnosed histologically from a sample of the lining.
- With simple enucleation, it seems that the recurrence rate may be from 25% to 60%.

In 2005, the World Health Organization renamed the lesion previously known as an odontogenic keratocyst as the keratocystic odontogenic tumor (KOT or KCOT).[1,2] The term odontogenic keratocyst was first used by Philipson in 1956[3] and its clinical and histologic features were confirmed by Browne in 1970 and 1971.[4,5] At that time, it was believed to be a benign, but potentially aggressive and recurrent, odontogenic cyst, and probably represented the lesion previously termed a primordial cyst.[6] Although most of these cysts were lined by parakeratinized epithelium, a few were orthokeratinized. Over the years, it has generally been agreed that the orthokeratinized versions have a lower incidence of recurrence than the parakeratinized version. As initially described, it was believed that the primitive nature of the epithelium may have a premalignant potential,[7] but this is now believed not to be true, and the incidence of malignant transformation is probably extremely low,[8] if it exists at all.

However, since its designation, some have believed that although it was designated as an odontogenic cyst, the lesion behaved more like a tumor.[9–11] The reasons for this belief include its clinical behavior, with a high recurrence rate after simple enucleation, the histologic appearance, and, more recently, the presence of tumor markers within the cyst. These markers consist of specifically proliferating cell nuclear antigen (PCNA), Ki67, BCE 2 sequence of the enzyme dihydrolipoyl acetyltransferase, matrix metalloproteinase (MMP) 2 and 9, and p53.[12–14] This combination of features led to the 2005 reclassification of this lesion, although a PubMed search of articles published since 2005 found that the lesion is still mostly referred to as an odontogenic keratocyst.[15] Even the term KCOT refers only to the parakeratinized version of the odontogenic keratocyst, and this leaves the orthokeratinized version of the cyst without a new designation. Until further reclassification, these orthokeratinized cysts are grouped with other benign odontogenic cysts.

## CAUSE

It is generally believed that these lesions originate from remnants of the dental lamina in the same way as the primordial cyst.[6] However, a tooth is generally not missing and, therefore, they are believed to originate from additional remnants of the lamina not involved in tooth formation. Alternatively, in some cases they may arise from the oral mucosa, particularly in the retromolar region, because daughter cysts are found between the oral mucosa and the cyst in the retromolar

Department of Oral and Maxillofacial Surgery, University of California San Francisco, Box 0440, Room C522, 521 Parnassus Avenue, San Francisco, CA 94143-0440, USA
E-mail address: tony.pogrel@ucsf.edu

Oral Maxillofacial Surg Clin N Am 25 (2013) 21–30
http://dx.doi.org/10.1016/j.coms.2012.11.003
1042-3699/13/$ – see front matter © 2013 Elsevier Inc. All rights reserved.

area.[16] Therefore, there may be 2 possible sites of origin of this lesion (**Fig. 1**).

## CLINICAL FEATURES

The clinical features associated with the KCOT show it to be a unilocular or multilocular radiolucency, occurring most frequently in the posterior mandible (the same site as the primordial cyst). It may or may not be associated with a missing tooth (usually not) (**Fig. 2**). Expansion of the buccal and lingual plates occurs late with this lesion (in contrast to the ameloblastoma), because it primarily tends to invade the marrow. However, it does cause some expansion of the lingual plate and can cause lingual plate perforation (**Fig. 3**). Inferior alveolar nerve involvement occurs late. Clinically, the lesion has a high recurrence potential if purely enucleated. Reports in the literature vary, but can show a recurrence rate of from 25% to 60% after local enucleation.[17–21] The

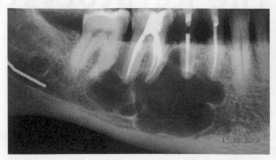

**Fig. 2.** A multilocular, multicystic KCOT of the right mandible not associated with a missing tooth. The complexity of the lesion contributes to difficulty in total removal.

reasons for this recurrence rate are believed to be 3-fold:

- They have a thin lining, which is friable, and portions are easily left behind.
- Daughter cysts occur beyond the visible margin of the lesion.
- Some of these lesions may originate from the oral mucosa and daughter cysts are seen between the oral mucosa and the cyst itself. Unless these lesions are removed, recurrence is likely (**Fig. 4**).

The basal cell nevus syndrome (also called Gorlin syndrome or Gorlin-Goltz syndrome) is a genetic condition with an autosomal-dominant inheritance pattern that includes a triad of KCOTs of the jaws,

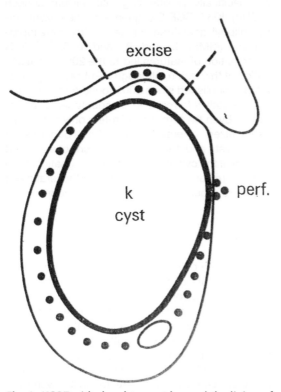

**Fig. 1.** KCOT with daughter cyst beyond the lining of the cyst and daughter cysts between the cyst and the alveolar mucosa. The area of alveolar mucosa that should be excised with the lesion is indicated. There is also a lingual perforation with associated daughter cysts. (*Adapted from* Bradley PF, Fisher AD. The cryosurgery of bone, an experimental and clinical assessment. Br J Oral Surg 1975;13:122; with permission.)

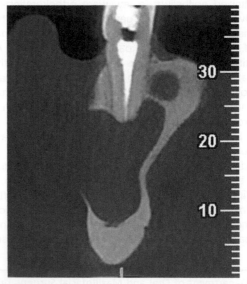

**Fig. 3.** A coronal cone-beam computed tomography scan showing a multilocular, multicystic KCOT, with lingual perforation and the inferior alveolar nerve embedded in the base of the lesion.

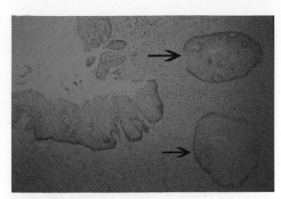

**Fig. 4.** Histologic specimen showing alveolar mucosa with daughter cysts (*arrows*) from KCOT between the alveolar mucosa and the cyst lining.

other skeletal abnormalities (often including bifid ribs, abnormalities in the length of the fingers and toes, frontal bossing, and calcification of the falx cerebri), as well as cutaneous manifestations such as basal cell carcinomas, palmar pitting of the hands, and other skin abnormalities.[22,23] Renal abnormalities and medulloblastomas in the newborn may also be manifestations of this condition. Whether sporadic or hereditary, most cases are related genetically and show aberrations in the hedgehog signaling pathway. The hedgehog signaling pathway involves a dynamic relationship between a series of tumor suppressor genes and oncogenes.

The basal cell carcinomas in this condition are atypical in that they occur on skin that is not sun-exposed and seem to be relatively benign and are often treated effectively with liquid nitrogen or silver nitrate sticks. Conversely, the KCOTs have often been believed to be particularly aggressive, with a tendency to recur, but in retrospect this may be more a question of the patient's developing additional lesions rather than recurrences of the previous ones. This condition seems most active up until the time that growth ceases, and patients often form many KCOTs during this period. Usually after growth ceases, the growth of the tumors slows considerably and new tumors develop more rarely. Because these tumors occur during the age of tooth development, it is often preferable to treat them by extensive marsupialization to expose the lining and allow the teeth to erupt, which seems to be successful and does not lead to a higher incidence of recurrence of the lesions. However, when this procedure is not appropriate, they can be managed in the usual way for KCOTs, with aggressive enucleation and curettage or even with peripheral, marginal, or segmental resection for particularly aggressive lesions.

## DIAGNOSIS

These tumors are normally diagnosed histologically from a sample of the lining. This diagnosis requires a surgical biopsy, and difficulties can arise when the cyst has been previously exposed or inflamed, when the lining tends to become thicker and less obviously parakeratinized. Diagnosis is normally made on permanent paraffin-stained sections, although attempts have been made to diagnosis it from frozen section so that definitive treatment can be performed at the same time as the biopsy. However, frozen sections of KCOTs have a high error rate of more than 35%, which may render this technique impractical.[21] Attempts have also been made to diagnose KCOTs from examination of a fluid aspirate. If subject to immediate histologic examination, keratin can often be seen under the microscope, and if the fluid is analyzed, the protein content (at <4.0 g/100 mL) is lower than that in serum (7.1 g/100 mL), which is also the protein content of a dentigerous cyst. It is also lower than that of an ameloblastoma, usually around 5.5 g/100 m.[24]

## TREATMENT

With simple enucleation, it seems that the recurrence rate may be from 25% to 60%. When treating the lesion as one would an ameloblastoma, including resection with 1-cm margins (this often necessitates a segmental resection), the recurrence rate can be virtually zero. However, this treatment may cause excessive morbidity. Therefore, although both of these techniques may be possible (simple enucleation in a patient with a limited life expectancy or segmental resection for a large lesion that has multiple cortical perforations), most of the search has been for an intermediate technique that gives an acceptable cure rate with an acceptable morbidity. Several of these techniques have been proposed.

### *Marsupialization or Decompression*

It was well known in the preantibiotic era that most dental cysts could be marsupialized and that this cured them. Marsupialization in its purest form consists of opening up the cyst to the oral cavity and suturing the cyst lining to the oral mucosa, creating a permanent opening into the cyst (**Fig. 5**). The cyst is, therefore, decompressed (most cysts grow by osmosis,[25] although the KCOT may also grow by bone resorption from prostaglandin production),[26] and decreases in size as new bone is laid down around it. This procedure was originally known as the Partsch I

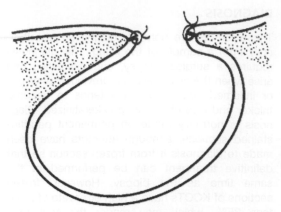

**Fig. 5.** Technique of marsupialization, with suturing of the cyst lining to the alveolar mucosa. (*From* Pogrel MA. Decompression and marsupialization as a treatment for the odontogenic keratocyst. Oral Maxillofac Surg Clin North Am 2003;15:416; with permission.)

technique.[27] With the advent of antibiotics, this technique was generally abandoned in favor of more definitive enucleation of dental cysts (the Partsch II technique).[28] However, the technique has been resurrected for the management of the KCOT. It is either used in its classic form of suturing the cyst lining to the oral mucosa (**Fig. 5**) or it is used more as a decompression technique, in which a smaller opening is made into the cyst, without suturing the lining and by use of a decompression tube of some kind (**Fig. 6**).[29–32] It has been noted in several studies that if this technique is used, the cyst decreases considerably in size and in most cases disappears completely radiographically.[33] It has also been

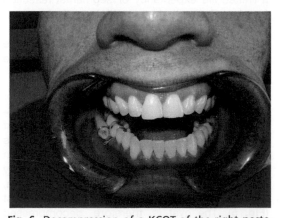

**Fig. 6.** Decompression of a KCOT of the right posterior mandible by means of a drainage tube wired to the first molar. The drainage tube often has to stay in place for 9 months to a year and be irrigated twice a day with normal saline by the patient, so it needs to be secure.

noted on biopsy of the lining that as the cyst decreases in size, the lining transforms from the thin parakeratinized lining to a thicker lining more resembling the oral mucosa.[34,35] It is not known whether this process happens by metaplasia in the KCOT lining or by overgrowth of more normal epithelium. In some techniques, it is recommended that the decompression be used for cure and complete resolution of the lesion (**Fig. 7**), whereas in others it is used to decompress the lesion and decrease its size, thicken the lining so that it is easier to remove, and when the cyst has decreased in size enough to be away from other structures (the inferior alveolar nerve and adjacent teeth), it can be enucleated. If this decompression technique is used for cure, then there does seem to be a 10% recurrence rate using the most currently available data.[36] If the decompression is used to decrease the size only, followed by more definitive enucleation of a lesion with a thicker lining, the long-term cure rate is undefined but may be higher.[37]

## Enucleation with Peripheral Ostectomy

If one accepts that the high recurrence rate after simple enucleation is caused by the presence of retained fragments of lining plus daughter cysts that are left behind, then it may be that removal of 1 to 2 mm of bone beyond the visible margin of the lesion is adequate to improve the cure rate. However, it is difficult to estimate how much bone to remove with a drill. This process is made easier by the use of a vital staining technique. Methylene blue or crystal violet (or any other vital stain) can be painted on the bony walls of the enucleated cyst and allowed to penetrate into the bone. The cavity is then washed out and any bone retaining the stain is removed with a drill (see **Fig. 8**). This process usually removes around 2 mm of bone in the marrow and about 1 mm of cortical bone. Good studies of the success rate of this technique do not exist, but it is believed to improve the cure rate.[38–40]

## Physicochemical Treatment

### Chemical treatment with Carnoy solution
The only chemical agent in use to increase the cure rate of the KCOT is Carnoy solution, and this remains controversial (**Fig. 9**). Originally used as a histologic fixative, it has been used clinically. Its classic ingredients are as follows:

Absolute alcohol: 6 mL
Chloroform: 3 mL
Ferric chloride: 1 g
Glacial acetic acid: 1 mL

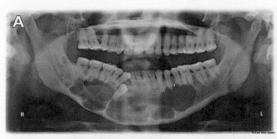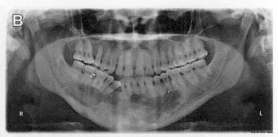

**Fig. 7.** (*A*) A large, multilocular KCOT of the mandible on initial presentation. (*B*) The same lesion 9 months later after biopsy, to establish the diagnosis, and insertion of 2 drainage tubes (seen on the radiograph) for decompression. The patient irrigated the drains twice daily with normal saline. The drains were removed after 1 year.

The most usual technique involves enucleation of the lesion followed by painting the sides of the cavity with Carnoy solution, leaving it in place for 5 minutes, and then washing out the cavity. After washing out, the cavity has brown, denatured bone on its wall. Some practitioners leave this bone in place, whereas others remove it with a drill to get down to normal bone. This technique generally involves a removal of 1 to 2 mm of bone. Carnoy solution is neurotoxic and chemically fixes the inferior alveolar or lingual nerves if it comes in contact with them for up to 2 minutes. The nerve should therefore be protected; bone wax can be used for protection of the inferior alveolar nerve.[41] The other issue with Carnoy solution, as originally formulated, is that it contains chloroform, now classified as a borderline carcinogen by the US Environmental Protection Agency (EPA) and as an outright carcinogen by the California EPA. For this reason, practitioners have used the solution without the chloroform, but cure rates with the modified Carnoy solution are not available. In addition, there is some debate as to whether or not Carnoy solution should be mixed fresh before use. Some investigators state that it should be

mixed fresh and used within 2 days, whereas others state that it can be left for several months. When supplied in the United States, the US Food and Drug Administration does approve it for up to 6 months. Results with the use of Carnoy solution show a low recurrence rate, in the order of 2.5%.[16,41–43]

### Physical treatment with cryotherapy

Freezing is known to cause cell death. However, to cause cell death (as in frostbite), freezing must be rapid and thawing should be slow, and temperatures less than –20°C must be achieved. The only commonly available agent that can achieve this temperature is liquid nitrogen, which boils at –196°C. Carbon dioxide and nitrous oxide both boil at temperatures high enough (–78.5°C and –89.7°C, respectively) that they cannot maintain –20°C consistently, particularly if there is any heat sink effect caused by adjacent blood vessels.[44] The technique using liquid nitrogen involves enucleation of the lesion followed by protection of the soft tissues with a combination of wooden tongue blades and dry gauze followed by treatment of the cyst cavity with the liquid

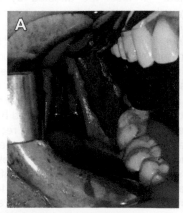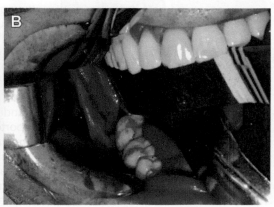

**Fig. 8.** (*A*) The cavity remaining after a cyst has been enucleated, and stained with methylene blue. (*B*) The same cavity after removing the methylene blue with a peripheral ostectomy using a pineapple-type bur.

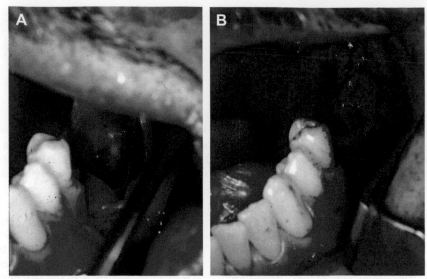

**Fig. 9.** (*A*) A KCOT of the left mandible enucleated. (*B*) The cavity subsequently treated with Carnoy solution. Note the brown appearance of the treated bone, which is often removed with a pineapple bur.

nitrogen (**Fig. 10**). For a cyst of less than 1.5 cm, the cyst cavity can be filled with a conductive medium such as KY jelly and a liquid nitrogen probe placed within it to freeze the whole mass (**Fig. 11**). For a larger cavity, the liquid nitrogen must be sprayed into the cavity, and for this, a long (about 20.3 cm [8 inches]) intravenous-type cannula is preferred, because it can be directed into any part of the cavity. The technique involves freezing the cavity walls until a frost forms (**Fig. 12**). The frost should be maintained for 1 minute with repeated sprays and then allowed to thaw. The thaw should be slow and natural, because this increases cell death by causing osmotic imbalance. Once it is thawed, the freeze is then normally repeated at least 1 more time for completeness in case any areas were missed on the first freeze.[45,46] Some practitioners prefer to give the area 3 freezes to be certain that no area is missed. Studies have shown that liquid nitrogen penetrates to at least 1.5 mm around the cavity.[47] If the inferior alveolar nerve is involved, the neuron degenerates, but the axon sheath is intact, and nerve regeneration is good, with most patients achieving at least some return of sensation and many patients achieving full return of sensation.[48] If teeth are affected by the cryotherapy, degenerative changes can occur in the pulpal tissues, but they often recover, and pulpal necrosis rarely needs treatment.[49] However, liquid nitrogen cryotherapy for bone does significantly weaken the bone until new osteogenesis occurs. This bone weakness reaches its maximum about 8 weeks after cryotherapy, and mandibular fractures around this time have been reported.[50] For this reason, we now recommend simultaneous cancellous marrow bone grafting for lesions grater than 3 to 4 cm to accelerate osteogenesis and decrease the chance of mandibular fracture.[51] Using this cryotherapy technique seems to be associated with a recurrence rate of around 10%, which is better than with enucleation alone.[52]

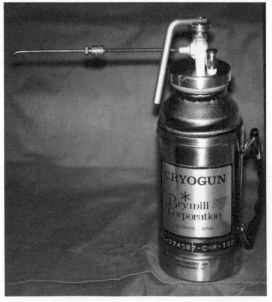

**Fig. 10.** A typical portable liquid nitrogen cryospray. The technology can also be used with a probe.

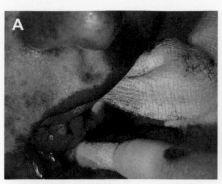
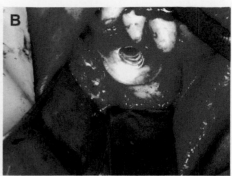

**Fig. 11.** (*A*) A smaller lesion treated with liquid nitrogen by the technique of filling the cavity with KY jelly and placing a liquid nitrogen probe in it and freezing the whole cavity. (*B*) The cryoprobe has been removed, showing the frozen KY jelly and surrounding bony walls of the cyst cavity. These frozen areas are allowed to thaw naturally and slowly and then the freeze is repeated. This technique can be used only for small lesions less than about 1.5 cm.

## Maxillary Tumors

Fortunately, keratocystic odontogenic tumors of the maxilla are unusual compared with those in the mandible (**Fig. 13**). However, there are potentially more issues and possible complications with maxillary lesions.

- The cortical bone is thinner so perforation can occur sooner.
- The presence of the maxillary sinus and nasal cavity mean that involvement of these areas can occur early.
- Radiographically, it is often difficult to separate the cyst from the maxillary sinus, even with CT scanning.
- Perforation into the pterygopalatine space can occur with lesions posteriorly placed in the maxilla and can make subsequent complete removal very difficult.

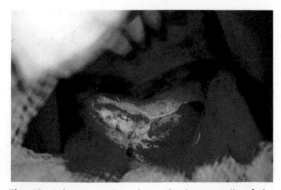

**Fig. 12.** A larger cavity where the bony walls of the cavity have been frozen by a liquid nitrogen spray. The frost is kept in place for 1 minute and is followed by a slow thawing process. This process can be repeated up to another 2 times.

For tumors of the anterior maxilla, treatment is essentially the same as for the mandible. As one moves more posteriorly in the maxilla, marsupialization is still a very viable option and the cavities normally shrink quickly. Unerupted teeth that have been displaced by the tumor may also start to erupt. This treatment may be particularly indicated in patients with Gorlin's syndrome. The cyst is normally decompressed or marsupialized into the buccal sulcus of the oral cavity, but theoretically it can be marsupialized into the maxillary sinus itself or even into the nasal cavity and these approaches have been described.

Lesions of the posterior maxilla, particularly those which are in proximity to the pterygomaxillary space may respond to marsupialization and decompression, but one should have a low threshold for carrying out a partial posterior maxillectomy with immediate reconstruction. An obturator is rarely necessary except for the largest lesions, and although this may mean the loss of teeth and alveolus, it stands the best chance of avoiding spread to the pterygomaxillary space. Carnoy's solution or liquid nitrogen can be used in smaller cysts which are completely surrounded by bony walls, but if there is any question of continuity with the sinus or nasal cavity, these modalities are best avoided and particularly in lesions which extend up to the orbital floor.

## THE AUTHOR'S CURRENT TECHNIQUE

Because none of these techniques seems to be associated with a zero recurrence rate, the author's current technique is as follows:

1. Obtain a tissue biopsy of the cyst. At the same time, a drainage tube is placed. This tube is normally made from either a piece of intravenous

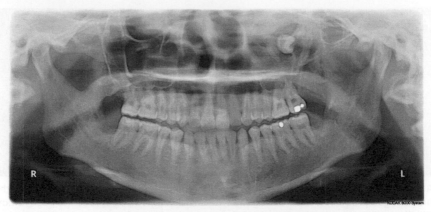

**Fig. 13.** Panorex of a KCOT of the left posterior maxilla, displacing the associated third molar. This KCOT needs to be imaged in 3 dimensions by means of a computed tomography scan and is probably treated by attempted decompression with a drainage tube followed by a partial posteroinferior maxillectomy and immediate reconstruction.

tubing or a pediatric feeding tube. They are similar to those advocated by Brodnum **(Fig. 6)**.[31]

2. If the diagnosis comes back as a KCOT, the drainage tube is left in place, the patient irrigates it twice a day with normal saline, and the size of the cyst is monitored radiographically every 3 months. The cysts normally start to regress quickly, and by 9 months to a year, have become smaller **(Fig. 7)**. If the biopsy shows a lesion other than KCOT, it is treated accordingly.

3. When the radiolucency has decreased to about 2 cm or less in diameter and is not in contact with adjacent teeth or the inferior alveolar nerve, it is enucleated and the cavity treated with liquid nitrogen cryotherapy given by means of a cryospray **(Figs. 11 and 12)**. If an adjacent tooth is still involved, it must be removed. At the same time as enucleation of the lesion, the overlying mucosa is excised to eliminate any daughter cysts between the overlying mucosa and the cyst. After cryotherapy, excellent soft tissue closure is required, because otherwise, wound breakdown is possible. A combination of vertical mattress sutures and simple interrupted sutures is preferred.

The author has been using this particular technique for 3.5 years and has treated 25 lesions in this manner. There have been no recurrences, although it is recognized that 3.5 years is an inadequate length of time to monitor these lesions. We recommend follow-up, primarily with panorex-type radiographs, every 6 months for 2 years, every year for 5 years, and every 2 years for 10 years in asymptomatic patients.

## REFERENCES

1. Philipsen HP. In: Barnes L, Eveson JW, Reichart P, et al, editors. World Health Organization classification of tumours. Pathology and genetics of head and neck tumours. Lyon (France): IARC; 2005. p. 306–7.
2. Reichart PA, Philipsen HP, Sciubba JJ. The new classification of head and neck tumours (WHO)–any changes? Oral Oncol 2006;42:757.
3. Philipsen HP. OM Keratocyster (Kolesten-Tomer). 1 Kaeberne. Tandialgebladet 1956;60:963 [in Danish].
4. Browne RM. The odontogenic keratocyst. Clinical aspects. Br Dent J 1970;128:225.
5. Browne RM. The odontogenic keratocyst. Histological features and their correlation with clinical behaviour. Br Dent J 1971;131:249.
6. Partridge M, Towers JF. The primordial cyst (odontogenic keratocyst): its tumour-like characteristics and behaviour. Br J Oral Maxillofac Surg 1987;25:271.
7. Browne RM, Gough NG. Malignant change in the epithelium lining odontogenic cysts. Cancer 1972; 29:1199.
8. Anand VK, Arrowood JP Jr, Krolls SO. Malignant potential of the odontogenic keratocyst. Otolaryngol Head Neck Surg 1994;111:124.
9. Shear M. The aggressive nature of the odontogenic keratocyst: is it a benign cystic neoplasm? Part 3. Immunocytochemistry of cytokeratin and other epithelial cell markers. Oral Oncol 2002;38:407.
10. Shear M. The aggressive nature of the odontogenic keratocyst: is it a benign cystic neoplasm? Part 2. Proliferation and genetic studies. Oral Oncol 2002; 38:323.
11. Shear M. The aggressive nature of the odontogenic keratocyst: is it a benign cystic neoplasm? Part 1. Clinical and early experimental evidence of aggressive behaviour. Oral Oncol 2002;38:219.

12. Slootweg PJ. p53 protein and Ki-67 reactivity in epithelial odontogenic lesions. An immunohistochemical study. J Oral Pathol Med 1995;24:393.

13. Barreto DC, Gomez RS, Bale AE, et al. PTCH gene mutations in odontogenic keratocysts. J Dent Res 2000;79:1418.

14. Cohen MM Jr. Nevoid basal cell carcinoma syndrome: molecular biology and new hypotheses. Int J Oral Maxillofac Surg 1999;28:216.

15. Bhargava D, Deshpande A, Pogrel MA. Keratocystic odontogenic tumour (KCOT)–a cyst to a tumour. Oral Maxillofac Surg 2012;16(2):163–70.

16. Stoelinga PJ. Long-term follow-up on keratocysts treated according to a defined protocol. Int J Oral Maxillofac Surg 2001;30:14.

17. Vedtofte P, Praetorius F. Recurrence of the odontogenic keratocyst in relation to clinical and histological features. A 20-year follow-up study of 72 patients. Int J Oral Surg 1979;8:412.

18. Brannon RB. The odontogenic keratocyst. A clinicopathologic study of 312 cases. Part I. Clinical features. Oral Surg Oral Med Oral Pathol 1976;42:54.

19. Pindborg JJ, Hansen J. Studies on odontogenic cyst epithelium. 2. Clinical and roentgenologic aspects of odontogenic keratocysts. Acta Pathol Microbiol Scand 1963;58:283.

20. Rud J, Pindborg JJ. Odontogenic keratocysts: a follow-up study of 21 cases. J Oral Surg 1969;27:323.

21. Guthrie D, Peacock ZS, Sadow P, et al. Preoperative incisional and intraoperative frozen section biopsy techniques have comparable accuracy in the diagnosis of benign intraosseous jaw pathology. J Oral Maxillofac Surg 2012;70(11):2566–72.

22. Scully C, Langdon J, Evans J. Marathon of eponyms; 7 Gorlin-Goltz syndrome (naevoid basal cell carcinoma syndrome). Oral Dis 2010;16:117–8.

23. Todd R, August M. Molecular approaches to the diagnosis of sporadic and naevoid basal cell carcinoma syndrome-associated odontogenic keratocysts. Oral Maxillofac Surg Clin North Am 2003;15: 447–61.

24. Toller PA. Protein substances in odontogenic cyst fluids. Br Dent J 1970;128:317.

25. Toller PA. The osmolality of fluids from cysts of the jaws. Br Dent J 1970;129:275.

26. Harris M. Odontogenic cyst growth and prostaglandin-induced bone resorption. Ann R Coll Surg Engl 1978; 60:85.

27. Partsch C. Über Kiefercysten. Deutsche Monatsschrift für Zahnheilkunde 1892;10:271 [in German].

28. Partsch CP. Zur Behandlung der Kiefercysten. Deutsche Monatsschrift für Zahnheilkunde 1910;28:252 [in German].

29. Ninomiya T, Kubota Y, Koji T, et al. Marsupialization inhibits interleukin-1alpha expression and epithelial cell proliferation in odontogenic keratocysts. J Oral Pathol Med 2002;31:526.

30. Eyre J, Zakrzewska JM. The conservative management of large odontogenic keratocysts. Br J Oral Maxillofac Surg 1985;23:195.

31. Brondum N, Jensen VJ. Recurrence of keratocysts and decompression treatment. A long-term follow-up of forty-four cases. Oral Surg Oral Med Oral Pathol 1991;72:265.

32. Marker P, Brondum N, Clausen PP, et al. Treatment of large odontogenic keratocysts by decompression and later cystectomy: a long-term follow-up and a histologic study of 23 cases. Oral Surg Oral Med Oral Pathol Oral Radiol Endod 1996;82:122.

33. Nakamura N, Mitsuyasu T, Mitsuyasu Y, et al. Marsupialization for odontogenic keratocysts: long-term follow-up analysis of the effects and changes in growth characteristics. Oral Surg Oral Med Oral Pathol Oral Radiol Endod 2002;94:543.

34. Pogrel MA, Jordan RC. Marsupialization as a definitive treatment for the odontogenic keratocyst. J Oral Maxillofac Surg 2004;62:651.

35. August M, Faquin WC, Troulis M, et al. Differentiation of odontogenic keratocysts from nonkeratinizing cysts by use of fine-needle aspiration biopsy and cytokeratin-10 staining. J Oral Maxillofac Surg 2000;58:935.

36. Pogrel MA. Decompression and marsupialization as definitive treatment for keratocysts–a partial retraction. J Oral Maxillofac Surg 2007;65:362.

37. August M, Faquin WC, Troulis MJ, et al. Dedifferentiation of odontogenic keratocyst epithelium after cyst decompression. J Oral Maxillofac Surg 2003; 61:678–83.

38. Kolokythas A, Fernandes RP, Pazoki A, et al. Odontogenic keratocyst: to decompress or not to decompress? A comparative study of decompression and enucleation versus resection/peripheral ostectomy. J Oral Maxillofac Surg 2007;65:640.

39. Sharif F, Oliver R, Sweet C, et al. Interventions for the treatment of keratocystic odontogenic tumours (KCOT, odontogenic keratocysts (OKC)). Cochrane Database Syst Rev 2010;(9):CD008464.

40. Irvine GH, Bowerman JE. Mandibular keratocysts: surgical management. Br J Oral Maxillofac Surg 1985;23:204.

41. Chapelle KA, Stoelinga PJ, de Wilde PC, et al. Rational approach to diagnosis and treatment of ameloblastomas and odontogenic keratocysts. Br J Oral Maxillofac Surg 2004;42:381.

42. Stoelinga PJ. The treatment of odontogenic keratocysts by excision of the overlying, attached mucosa, enucleation, and treatment of the bony defect with Carnoy solution. J Oral Maxillofac Surg 2005;63:1662.

43. Voorsmit RA, Stoelinga PJ, van Haelst UJ. The management of keratocysts. J Maxillofac Surg 1981;9:228.

44. Bradley PF, Fisher AD. The cryosurgery of bone. An experimental and clinical assessment. Br J Oral Surg 1975;13:111.

45. Pogrel MA. The management of lesions of the jaws with liquid nitrogen cryotherapy. J Calif Dent Assoc 1995;23:54.

46. Schmidt BL, Pogrel MA. The use of enucleation and liquid nitrogen cryotherapy in the management of odontogenic keratocysts. J Oral Maxillofac Surg 2001;59:720.

47. Pogrel MA, Regezi JA, Fong B, et al. Effects of liquid nitrogen cryotherapy and bone grafting on artificial bone defects in minipigs: a preliminary study. Int J Oral Maxillofac Surg 2002;31:296.

48. Schmidt BL, Pogrel MA. Neurosensory changes after liquid nitrogen cryotherapy. J Oral Maxillofac Surg 2004;62:1183.

49. Gordon NC, Laskin DM. The effects of local hypothermia on odontogenesis. J Oral Surg 1979;37:235.

50. Fisher AD, Williams DF, Bradley PF. The effect of cryosurgery on the strength of bone. Br J Oral Surg 1978;15:215.

51. Salmassy DA, Pogrel MA. Liquid nitrogen cryosurgery and immediate bone grafting in the management of aggressive primary jaw lesions. J Oral Maxillofac Surg 1995;53:784.

52. Schmidt BL. The use of liquid nitrogen cryotherapy in the management of the odontogenic keratocyst. Oral Maxillofac Surg Clin North Am 2003;15:393.

# The Diagnosis and Management of Parotid Disease

Eric R. Carlson, DMD, MD[a],*, David E. Webb, Maj, USAF, DC[b]

## KEYWORDS

- Fine-needle aspiration biopsy • Superficial parotidectomy • Partial superficial parotidectomy
- Extracapsular dissection

## KEY POINTS

- The diagnosis and management of patients with disease of the parotid gland represents a formidable discipline in oral and maxillofacial surgery.
- Disease of the parotid gland is represented by a diverse array of diagnoses, ranging from acute infection to malignant neoplastic disease with facial nerve palsy.
- A specific and regimented approach to such disease is necessary so as to properly diagnose and manage the disease in a timely fashion.
- Evaluation of patients with a parotid lesion should result in the development of a differential diagnosis that includes neoplastic and nonneoplastic entities.

## INTRODUCTION

Evaluation of patients with a parotid lesion should result in the development of a differential diagnosis that includes neoplastic and nonneoplastic entities. The primary exercise in the initial evaluation of a patient with a parotid swelling, therefore, is to distinguish neoplastic from nonneoplastic processes and to initiate the exercise of proper diagnosis and treatment.[1] Salivary gland tumors as a whole are rare compared with the overall incidence of head and neck tumors. Overall, salivary gland tumors vary worldwide from about 0.4 to 13.5 cases per 100,000 people in the population.[2] The parotid gland is the most common site of occurrence of salivary gland tumors, generally comprising 60% to 75% of all salivary gland tumors in large series (**Table 1**).[3–6] The most common benign tumor of the parotid gland and the most common salivary gland tumor overall is the pleomorphic adenoma. The most common

malignant tumor of the parotid gland is the mucoepidermoid carcinoma. Most nonneoplastic salivary gland swellings represent acute or chronic infections of these glands.[7] Although any of the major or minor salivary glands can become infected, these conditions most commonly occur in the parotid and submandibular glands, with the sublingual and minor salivary glands rarely becoming infected. From an etiologic standpoint, these infections are caused by a diverse number of bacterial, mycobacterial, viral, fungal, or parasitic organisms, or occasionally by immunologically mediated mechanisms. Moreover, an equally diverse number of risk factors may predispose patients to parotid infections (**Box 1**). An assessment has been reported of the relative frequency of neoplastic versus nonneoplastic disease of the major salivary glands, including the parotid gland. In this study, the investigators evaluated 140 parotidectomy specimens, 102

[a] Department of Oral and Maxillofacial Surgery, University of Tennessee Graduate School of Medicine and the University of Tennessee Cancer Institute, 1930 Alcoa Highway, Suite 335, Knoxville, TN 37920, USA; [b] David Grant Medical Center, 60th Dental Squadron, 101 Bodin Circle, Travis Air Force Base, CA, USA
* Corresponding author.
*E-mail address:* ecarlson@mc.utmck.edu

Oral Maxillofacial Surg Clin N Am 25 (2013) 31–48
http://dx.doi.org/10.1016/j.coms.2012.10.001
1042-3699/13/$ – see front matter © 2013 Elsevier Inc. All rights reserved.

**Table 1**
**Frequency of parotid tumors amongst salivary gland tumors**

| References | Number of Salivary Gland Cases | Number of Parotid Neoplasms (%) | Number of Benign/Malignant Parotid Neoplasms (%) |
|---|---|---|---|
| Ellis et al,[3] 1991 | 13,749 | 8222 (59.8) | 5566 (67.7)/2656 (32.3) |
| Eveson and Cawson[4] 1985 | 2410 | 1756 (72.9) | 1498 (85.3)/258 (14.7) |
| Spiro[5] 1986 | 2807 | 1965 (70) | 1342 (68.3)/623 (31.7) |
| Ito et al,[6] 2005 | 496 | 336 (67.7) | 256 (76.2)/80 (23.8) |

(73%) of which showed neoplastic disease and 38 (27%) specimens showed nonneoplastic entities.[8] In this study, the investigators also examined 110 submandibular gland excisions, 17 (15%) of which were performed for neoplastic disease and 93 (85%) of which were performed for nonneoplastic disease. When examining a patient with a parotid swelling, therefore, the likelihood of a neoplastic process should be highly considered, because it is more likely than when examining a patient with a submandibular swelling.

## INITIAL EVALUATION AND GENERAL CONCEPTS
### History

The initial evaluation of a patient with a parotid gland swelling must begin with a comprehensive history and physical examination, which should primarily distinguish infectious/obstructive processes from neoplastic processes. Historical elements that must be considered during this initial evaluation include whether the examination is being performed in an inpatient or outpatient setting; the patient's specific symptoms and their chronicity; and the possible presence of systemic disease. A patient with acute parotid swelling who is examined in an intensive care unit setting after surgery, for example, might be experiencing a parotitis. By contrast, a patient with a 10-year history of parotid swelling who is being examined in an outpatient setting might be experiencing a parotid neoplasm. The setting in which this initial evaluation occurs provides valuable information as to the cause of a parotid swelling, including a parotitis. For example, the microbiological cause and treatment of a community-acquired parotitis is different from that of a hospital-acquired parotitis. The clinician may begin to disclose important information as to the cause of the parotitis based on the setting in which they are examining the patient. In general terms, gram-positive organisms are more commonly encountered in community-acquired infections, whereas gram-negative

organisms are more commonly encountered in hospital-acquired infections.

Symptoms being experienced by patients with parotid enlargement may further divulge their disease state and also qualify its magnitude. The presence of a painful swelling, particularly prandial pain, or pain during eating, may suggest a diagnosis of sialolithiasis. However, prandial pain is not pathognomonic of a diagnosis of sialolithiasis, because parotitis unrelated to sialolithiasis may also present in this way. Moreover, some patients with malignant tumors of the parotid gland complain of pain such that early discovery of such malignancies is of paramount importance. The patient's perception of the expression of purulence from the salivary duct should be ascertained during the history. Clearly, the greater the magnitude of purulent infection noted on physical examination, the greater the likelihood that admission to the hospital and incision and drainage are necessary. In addition, the presence of a significant volume of purulence at the opening of a salivary duct may point to the value of obtaining special imaging studies for proper patient management.

Obtaining information regarding the presence of comorbid systemic disease and therapeutic medications is an important aspect of the history taking of all patients regardless of their chief complaint. With regard to patients in particular with parotid swellings, inquiring as to the presence of diabetes, HIV/AIDS, and recent surgery may permit the disclosure of nonmodifiable, relatively nonmodifiable, and modifiable predisposing features of parotitis (see **Box 1**).

### Physical Examination

The performance of a physical examination follows the history taking and may permit the clinician to distinguish an infectious/obstructive process from a neoplastic process (**Fig. 1**). In particular, extraoral inspection and palpation of the parotid swelling may determine the presence or absence of tenderness, erythema, and warmth. Intraoral inspection and palpation may identify purulence

---

**Box 1**
**Risk factors associated with parotid gland infections**

*Nonmodifiable risk factors*

Advanced age of patient

*Relatively nonmodifiable risk factors*

Anorexia nervosa/bulimia

Congestive heart failure

Cushing disease

Cystic fibrosis

Diabetes mellitus

Human immunodeficiency virus (HIV)/AIDS

Hepatic failure

Renal failure

S/P radiation therapy to parotid gland

*Modifiable risk factors*

Dehydration

Malnutrition

Medications

    Anticholinergics

    Antihistamines

    Antihypertensives

    Antisialagogues

    Barbiturates

    Chemotherapeutic agents

    Diuretics

    Phenothiazines

    Tricyclic antidepressants

Oral infection

Sialolithiasis

---

or a stone at the Stenson's duct. Intraoral examination and inspection of the quality and quantity of expressed parotid saliva is an essential aspect of the physical examination (**Fig. 2**). Examination of the soft palate and the lateral pharynx is indicated so as to determine if the deep lobe of the parotid gland might contain tumor. In addition, an evaluation of the cervical lymph nodes may give the clinician the impression of no adenopathy, inflammatory adenopathy, or metastatic adenopathy related to a parotid malignancy. Specifically, inflammatory lymph nodes may show tenderness and a compressible nature on physical examination, whereas metastatic lymph nodes are more likely to be nontender and indurated on physical examination. Further, the integrity of the facial

nerve should be assessed in all patients with parotid swellings (**Fig. 3**). At the time of the history and physical examination of a patient with a parotid swelling, a decision should be made as to whether basic imaging with a panoramic radiograph is indicated. This radiograph is occasionally able to show the presence of an intraglandular or extraglandular stone associated with the parotid gland (**Fig. 4**). Panoramic radiographs should be obtained in patients with a diffuse parotid swelling suggestive of inflammatory disease so as to rule out the presence of a sialolith.

## Laboratory Investigation

The usefulness of obtaining blood tests in a patient with parotid disease largely centers on the investigation for dehydration and the magnitude of leukocytosis in the case of a parotitis identified on physical examination. The serum electrolytes, particularly sodium, osmolarity, and white blood cell count, should be scrutinized in all patients with a suppurative parotitis, but specifically in those patients admitted to the hospital, including postoperative patients and those patients admitted to an intensive care unit. Intravenous fluid resuscitation as well as antibiotic administration represents first-line therapy for inpatients with a suppurative parotitis. On occasion, an outpatient requires admission to the hospital for similar therapy for parotitis. Under such circumstances, the magnitude of the leukocytosis, if present, as well as the general appearance of the patient as noted on physical examination, assists the surgeon in determining if an admission to the hospital is indicated. A stat Gram stain with aerobic and anaerobic culture and sensitivity of expressed pus at Stenson's duct should be obtained in all patients with a suppurative parotitis, and preferably before initiating antibiotic therapy.

## Imaging

The results of the history and physical examination lead to a decision as to whether a sophisticated imaging study is required to assist in the diagnosis and treatment planning. Computed tomography (CT) is indicated in the assessment of patients with parotid swellings related to infectious disease (**Fig. 5**A) as well as patients with suspected parotid neoplasms (see **Fig. 5**B). CT scans in both types of patients anatomically define the location of a neoplasm in preparation for tumor surgery or quantify the magnitude of infection and possible abscess in the case of an infectious process. If significant salivary infection is noted on imaging studies, a decision can be made to perform incision and drainage of the parotid abscess.

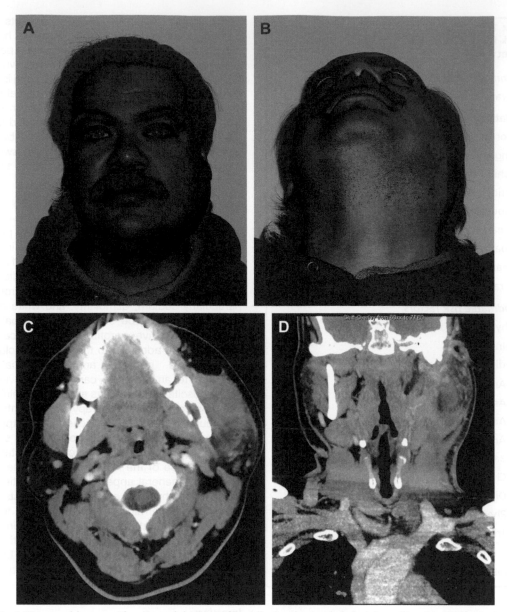

**Fig. 1.** A 39-year-old man with a 3-week history of rapidly developing left facial swelling (*A, B*). Physical examination revealed diffuse swelling of the left parotid gland and trismus with cervical adenopathy. Axial (*C*) and coronal (*D*) computed tomography (CT) scans supported a diagnosis of acute parotitis. The patient was treated with antibiotics and the process resolved. This patient is compared with a 64-year-old man with a 2-year history of left facial swelling (*E, F*). Physical examination revealed a discrete mass of the superior aspect of the left parotid gland. Axial (*G*) and coronal (*H*) CT scans showed an enhancing mass of the left superficial lobe of the parotid gland that abutted the mandibular condyle. A left superficial parotidectomy was performed, which identified mucoepidermoid carcinoma.

Moreover, CT scans anatomically define the location of an intraglandular or extraglandular stone in the case of sialolithiasis. Magnetic resonance imaging (MRI) scans may be substituted for CT scans according to the preference of the surgeon. One particular benefit of MRI scans is the ability to suggest a likely diagnosis of pleomorphic adenoma of a salivary gland when a hyperintense and well-localized mass is noted on T2-weighted images.

Once imaging studies are obtained, the surgeon may wish to perform a fine-needle aspiration biopsy (FNAB) for additional diagnostic information or the surgeon may elect to proceed directly

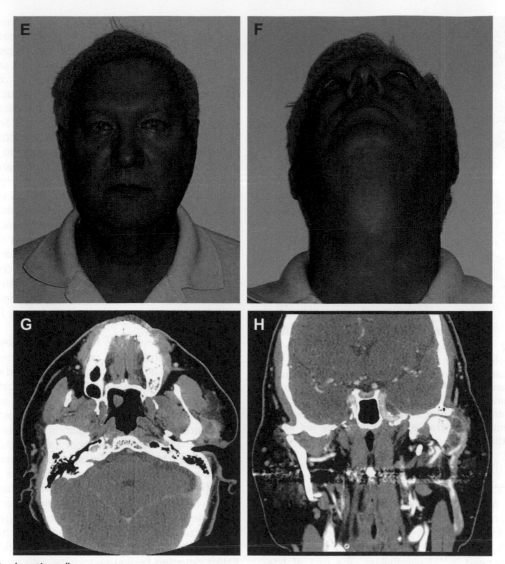

**Fig. 1.** (*continued*)

with surgical intervention associated with the pathologic process of the parotid gland, whether it is suspected to represent a neoplastic or non-neoplastic process. When an FNAB is preferred, it can be performed in the office or with imaging guidance.

## TECHNIQUES INVOLVED IN THE DIAGNOSIS AND MANAGEMENT OF PAROTID DISEASE
### FNAB

The parotid glands can show a wide range of pathologic changes, which can be challenging to properly characterize exclusively by clinical features. Benign lesions may resemble malignant lesions and vice versa. No single diagnostic modality is accepted unequivocally as the definitive approach

to parotid disease.[9] Although it is generally accepted that FNAB is useful in the preoperative setting, the accuracy is highly dependent on both operator experience and the diagnostic skills of the cytopathologist. Results of the FNAB must be considered by the surgeon in the global context, correlating the patient's history, physical examination, and imaging studies.[9] FNAB is generally considered a rapid, simple, inexpensive and complication-free method of initial diagnosis of head and neck lesions, including parotid swellings (**Fig. 6**). It is of value in providing a sample of pus for Gram stain, culture, and sensitivity in the case of a suspected suppurative parotitis or providing a sample for cytologic diagnosis in the case of a suspected parotid neoplasm. Fine-needle aspiration of a parotid neoplasm has the

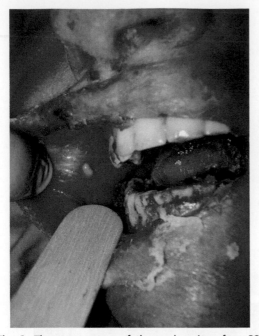

**Fig. 2.** The appearance of the oral cavity of an 88-year-old woman admitted to the intensive care unit after abdominal surgery. Physical examination identified an enlarged right parotid gland and pus at the opening of the Stenson's duct. This patient is clearly dehydrated, as noted by the dry oral mucosa. The patient's postoperative dehydrated state led to the parotitis.

distinct advantage of not seeding the overlying skin, which would otherwise occur if open biopsy or a core biopsy had been performed of a parotid neoplasm. If skin is seeded with tumor, subsequent proper surgical management is less likely to succeed.[10,11] Nevertheless, the role of fine-needle aspiration has not been universally accepted and its use remains controversial.[12] Batsakis and colleagues[13] have argued that most parotid masses require surgical removal such that FNAB has no meaningful influence on the management of patients with parotid disease. Nonetheless, fine-needle aspiration has been described as being part of a triple assessment of a parotid gland swelling, which also includes a clinical examination and an imaging study when deemed appropriate.[14] These investigators also pointed out that FNAB helps to avoid unnecessary surgery in many cases. Heller and colleagues[15] reported that cytologic assessment altered patient management in greater than one-third of cases, most commonly in the avoidance of surgery.

When considering an FNAB of a discrete parotid mass that was identified on physical examination and further defined on an imaging study, the surgeon should also consider the information that they wish to glean from such an aspiration. From the surgeon's standpoint, perhaps the most important piece of information that should be sought is the neoplastic character of the discrete mass, specifically, whether the tumor is benign or malignant (**Fig. 7**). This information not only permits the surgeon to discuss this finding with the patient during an informed consent process but it also permits the surgeon to offer the patient a neck dissection if a malignancy is identified on the needle biopsy. From a practical standpoint, the diagnosis of benign versus malignant is the only important piece of information that is required. The specific type of benign or malignant tumor is probably not required of the cytologist interpreting the needle aspiration, because surgical treatment is not likely to change within the categories of benign versus malignant disease. To this end, it is important to review the reported sensitivity and specificity of FNAB (**Table 2**).

Atula and colleagues[12] reviewed 438 FNABs of the parotid gland in 365 patients and compared these with final histopathology of the parotid specimens, and also assessed the outcome of patients who were not operated. Two hundred and seventeen FNABs from 191 parotid lesions in 175 patients were obtained from parotid glands that were not operated with follow-up of hospital records over a period of 2 to 9 years available to the investigators. Two hundred and seven FNABs were taken from 188 primary parotid tumors in 187 patients in whom histopathology of the parotid tumor was available to the investigators. The cytology was categorized as either nonneoplastic, benign neoplastic, possibly malignant, and malignant. FNAB detected benign neoplasms with an accuracy of 78% in this study, whereas the accuracy in detecting malignant tumors was 84%. A false-negative rate of 45% for malignancies was established in this study. Fifty percent of the 22 FNABs that were classified as possibly malignant were benign tumors by histopathology. Cytology was benign in 196 (90%) FNABs of 217 not confirmed by histology. During the follow-up of 2 to 9 years, only 2 patients proved to have malignant tumors amongst the group of cytologically benign lesions. The investigators concluded their study by indicating that FNAB should be used as a building block in the diagnosis of parotid lesions. They also concluded that the cytologic findings must correlate with the clinical picture, and a report of normal tissue or cystic fluid from a parotid lesion should not necessarily be accepted as a final diagnosis.

Ali and colleagues[16] retrospectively reviewed 129 patients with parotid lesions who had

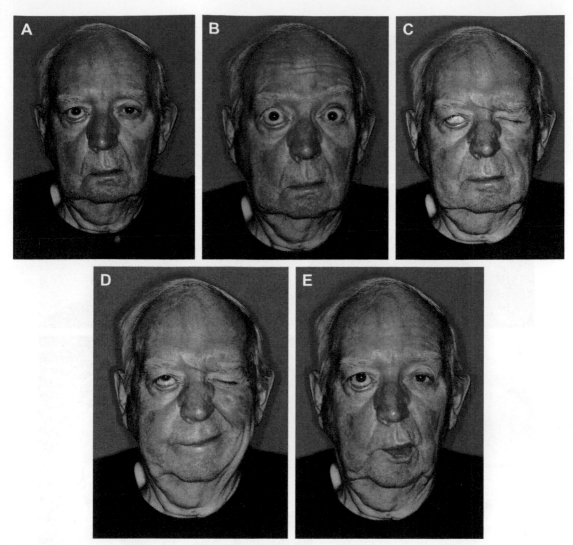

**Fig. 3.** An 83-year-old man with a 6-month history of a right paralytic ectropion (*A*). Physical examination also identified a right parotid mass. A complete right facial nerve palsy was noted on examination, including the temporal branch (*B*), the zygomatic branch (*C*), the buccal branch (*D*), and the marginal mandibular branch (*E*).

undergone parotid surgery and for whom histologic assessment of their parotid disease was available. There were 98 benign lesions diagnosed and 31 malignant tumors diagnosed. The sensitivity of the FNAB was 84%, the specificity was 98%, and the accuracy was 94%. The FNAB result was nondiagnostic in 5 (3.8%) cases. The investigators of this study correctly typed pleomorphic adenoma in 73 of 77 (95%) cases. Of the 98 benign histologic diagnoses in this study, 86 (88%) were correctly typed. Fourteen of 16 (87.5%) cases of mucoepidermoid carcinoma were correctly typed, and 4 of 4 cases of adenoid cystic carcinoma were correctly typed in this study. Of the 31 cases of malignant parotid tumors in this study, 24 (88%) were correctly typed. The investigators indicated

that FNAB plays an important role in the accurate diagnosis of parotid tumors. They pointed out that the accurate preoperative differentiation of these tumors may prepare the surgeon and patient for an appropriate surgical procedure. Christensen and colleagues[17] found that a correct subtyping of a benign salivary gland lesion was achieved in 97% of their cases, and the accurate diagnosis of a malignancy was achieved in 71% of their cases. Layfield[18] pointed out that one of the most difficult lesions within the salivary glands to accurately diagnose with FNAB is the mucoepidermoid carcinoma, indicating that these neoplasms are both overdiagnosed and underdiagnosed. Mucoepidermoid carcinomas can be cytologically divided into low-grade and

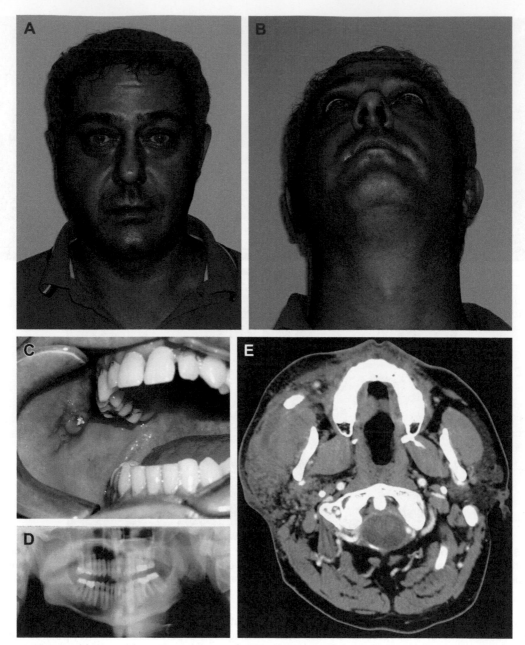

**Fig. 4.** A 43-year-old man with a 12-year history of right parotid swelling (*A, B*). Physical examination identified diffuse indurated swelling of the right parotid gland and a sialolith at the right Stenson's duct (*C*). The panoramic radiograph (*D*) showed the sialolith to be superimposed on the crown of tooth 2. The axial computed tomography scan showed the sialolith as well as an ectacic Stenson's duct proximal to the stone, which indicates obstruction of salivary flow (*E*).

high-grade neoplasms. Low-grade mucoepidermoid carcinomas may be difficult to separate from mucous retention cysts. High-grade mucoepidermoid carcinomas may be cytologically difficult to separate from squamous cell carcinomas and adenocarcinomas of the parotid glands.

Zbaren and colleagues[19] analyzed and compared the value of FNAB and frozen section in the assessment of parotid tumors. The investigators performed a chart review and cross-sectional analysis of 838 patients with previously untreated parotid pathologies who were operated on between 1987 and 2007 in their institution. A preoperative FNAB was performed in 426 patients and a frozen-section analysis was performed in 166 patients. One hundred and ten patients were

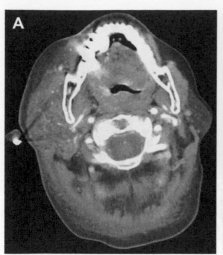
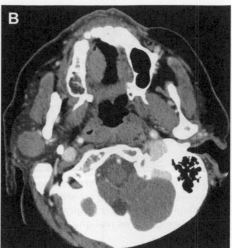

**Fig. 5.** (*A*) An axial CT scan showing signs consistent with an inflammatory process of the right parotid gland. The gland is enlarged and the vasculature is prominent within the gland. Mild fat stranding is also appreciated in the region of the right parotid gland. (*B*) An axial CT scan showing a discrete enhancing mass of the right parotid gland that is indicative of neoplastic disease.

enrolled in the study. The sensitivity, specificity, and accuracy of FNAB were 74%, 88%, and 79%, respectively. The sensitivity, specificity, and accuracy of frozen section were 93%, 95% and 94%, respectively. The histologic tumor type was correctly diagnosed by FNAB and frozen section in 27 of 42 (64%) and 39 of 42 (93%) benign tumors, respectively, and 24 of 68 (35%) and 49 of 68 (72%) malignant tumors, respectively.

The investigators summarized their study by identifying the superiority of frozen section over FNAB in detecting malignancy and tumor typing. They recommended frozen-section analysis for the determination of the histologic subtype or grade in planning the extent of surgery of malignant parotid tumors. These investigators indicted that FNAB is useful in avoiding surgery, in the case of inflammatory lesions, and in limiting

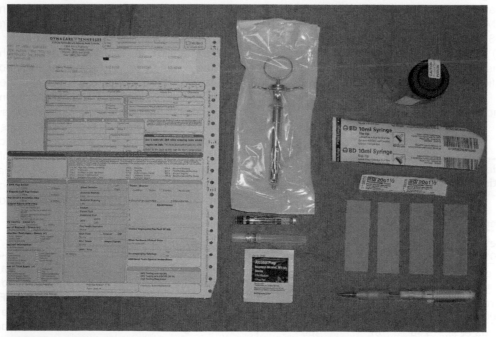

**Fig. 6.** The armamentarium for an FNAB of the parotid gland. A 20-gauge or smaller needle is used to avoid seeding of the tissue bed, which would otherwise occur if a larger needle (18-gauge) were used.

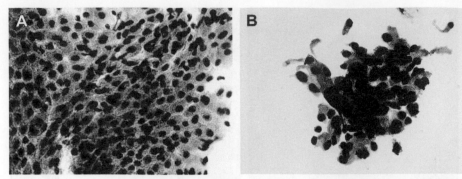

**Fig. 7.** Cytology of a benign tumor of the parotid gland (*A*) and a malignant tumor of the parotid gland (*B*). The benign tumor shows cytologic order where the cells form a honeycomb appearance, whereas the malignant tumor shows cytologic disorder. The surgical usefulness of the FNAB is that the surgeon proceeds with a provisional diagnosis of benign versus malignant without the need for a more specific diagnosis.

surgical procedures, in the case of benign parotid tumors.

Bartels and colleagues[20] established the sensitivity, specificity, and accuracy of imaging and FNAB, alone or in combination, in distinguishing benign from malignant parotid lesions. A retrospective study of all patients with parotid masses referred to their center was performed. Five hundred and eighty-six patients were identified, of whom 48 patients met all of the necessary criteria for inclusion in their study, including a parotid lesion of any histologic origin, FNAB results with sufficient cells, available final surgical pathologic results, and adequate preoperative imaging studies available for review. Thirteen of the patients were imaged with CT scans and 35 with MRI. Pathologic examination revealed that 23 (48%) of the lesions were malignant and 25 (52%) were benign. The evaluation of the parotid lesions with FNAB alone resulted in a sensitivity, specificity, and accuracy of 83%, 86%, and 85%, respectively. The sensitivity, specificity, and accuracy of CT alone were 100%, 42%, and 69%, respectively. The sensitivity, specificity,

and accuracy of MRI alone were 88%, 77%, and 83%, respectively. The sensitivity, specificity, and accuracy of MRI combined with FNAB were 88%, 94%, and 91%, respectively. The sensitivity, specificity, and accuracy of CT combined with FNAB were 83%, 86%, and 85%, respectively. The investigators concluded that imaging and FNAB are comparable in their ability to correctly identify malignant parotid lesions preoperatively and that combining the 2 modalities yields no advantage in terms of sensitivity, specificity, and accuracy of a malignant diagnosis. Moreover, the investigators pointed out that many patients with a parotid mass do not require anything more than a careful history and physical examination for management of a well-circumscribed, mobile, slowly growing mass. They indicated that preoperative testing rarely changes the need for or nature of the operation. In instances of an atypical history, a fixed or poorly defined mass, or if the potential for facial nerve involvement was high, the additional testing to determine anatomic boundaries or the risk of malignancy may be useful in surgical planning and patient counseling. The results of this study suggested that MRI is the first test of choice, because it was as effective as FNAB at confirming the suspicion of malignancy, and the MRI can also provide detailed anatomic information about the extent of the primary tumor as well as the adjacent lymph nodes.

### Superficial Parotidectomy

The standard operation for the removal of a tumor of the superficial lobe of the parotid gland is the time-honored superficial parotidectomy (**Fig. 8**). As part of this surgery, the superficial lobe of the parotid gland is removed with the tumor and the entire course of the facial nerve is intentionally dissected and preserved, unless it is directly

**Table 2**
**Statistical results of FNABs of parotid lesions**

| References | Number of Cases | Sensitivity (%) | Specificity (%) |
|---|---|---|---|
| Ali et al,[16] 2011 | 129 | 84 | 98 |
| Bartels et al,[20] 2000 | 48 | 83 | 86 |
| Zbaren et al,[19] 2008 | 426 | 74 | 88 |
| Zurrida et al,[10] 1993 | 246 | 62 | 100 |

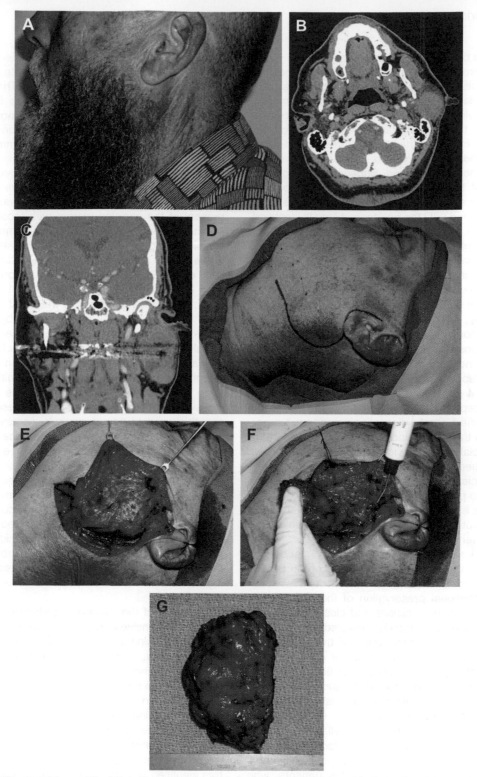

**Fig. 8.** A 59-year-old man (*A*) with an 8-year history of a left parotid mass. His beard had interfered with his frequent self-examination as a result of the lack of shaving. The recent onset of pain in the area led to his seeking consultation. Axial (*B*) and coronal (*C*) CT scans revealed a heterogeneous mass within most of the superficial lobe of the left parotid gland. A preoperative FNAB suggested the presence of a benign tumor. A left superficial parotidectomy was performed with a modified Blair incision (*D*). The dissection included the identification of the parotid capsule (*E*). The main trunk of the facial nerve was identified with the use of a nerve stimulator and the specimen was elevated off the full extent of the facial nerve (*F*). The pseudocapsule of the tumor remained intact as it was elevated off the nerve. The superficial parotidectomy specimen (*G*) was processed with permanent sections and carcinoma ex-pleomorphic adenoma was identified. The greater auricular nerve was sacrificed as part of this superficial parotidectomy.

invaded by the tumor. The approach to the superficial parotidectomy is typically with the modified Blair incision. The skin flap is elevated in a plane superficial to the parotid capsule. The sternocleidomastoid muscle is identified and the posterior edge of the parotid gland is separated from the muscle. Inferiorly, the platysma muscle is divided, and superior dissection is performed toward the tail of the parotid gland. Superiorly, the posterior edge of the parotid gland is sharply separated from the auricular cartilage. This sharp dissection is continued until the pointer cartilage is identified. Although the pointer cartilage does point to the main trunk of the facial nerve, the nerve is located more deeply in this region. A nerve stimulator is used at this time so as to initiate the process of identifying the main trunk of the facial nerve. The posterior belly of the digastric muscle is identified inferiorly, and blunt dissection is performed in a superior direction so as to identify the junction of the posterior belly of the digastric muscle and the sternocleidomastoid muscle. The main trunk of the facial nerve is predictably located approximately 4 mm superior to this junction and at the same depth as this junction. Once the main trunk is identified, careful dissection is performed superficial to this nerve, and the bifurcation of the temporofacial and cervicofacial trunks is noted. Continued dissection of the deep surface of the superficial lobe and pseudocapsule of the parotid tumor is performed, the entire course of the facial nerve is exposed, and the entire superficial lobe of the parotid gland is removed. The specimen is thereafter delivered.

The superficial parotidectomy specimen includes the entire superficial lobe of the parotid gland and tumor, with a resultant full dissection and intentional preservation of the facial nerve. Marginal tumor excisions and close margins are encountered and frankly expected in the region of the preserved main trunk of the facial nerve and its branches. The status of close margins has been studied extensively, particularly with regard to recurrence of the parotid tumor. Moreover, the status of the pseudocapsule that separates the tumor from the margin of the specimen has received due scrutiny as well. Ghosh and colleagues[21] have assessed risk factors for recurrence of marginally excised parotid pleomorphic adenomas. They reviewed 394 patients who underwent parotidectomy, of whom 274 had a diagnosis of pleomorphic adenoma. A total of 160 patients had an adequate cuff of tissue (several millimeters) surrounding the tumor, whereas 114 patients were considered to have a marginal clearance around their tumors and were therefore believed to be at risk for recurrence. Eighty-three of the 114 patients were included in the study because complete records were available for retrospective study. The overall recurrence rate in these patients was 6.0% (5 patients). Of the 5 recurrences, 3 tumors were noted to be widely present at the excision margin, 1 tumor was widely present within 1 mm of the margin, and 1 tumor showed a margin greater than 1 mm. This last case experienced tumor spillage at the time of surgery. The investigators compared the cases in which tumor was widely present at the excision margin with those cases in which tumor was present within 1 mm of the excision margin. The recurrence rate was 17.6% in the former group and 1.8% in the latter group. In 33 of the 83 cases (39.8%), the surgeon considered that the tumor was adherent to 1 or more branches of the main trunk of the facial nerve. In 91% of these cases, it was possible by careful dissection to avoid having tumor present at the excision margin. The investigators concluded by indicating that the adequacy of excision of pleomorphic adenomas depends primarily on the presence or absence or tumor cells at the surgical excision margin. The microscopic presence of any thickness of pseudocapsule containing the tumor translates to low risk of recurrence.

McGurk and colleagues[22] similarly examined the clinical significance of the tumor pseudocapsule in the treatment of parotid pleomorphic adenomas by superficial parotidectomy. Their incidence of 2% recurrence led to their conclusion that careful dissection close to a pleomorphic adenoma need not lead to a high incidence of recurrence and that in practice the microinvasion of the capsule by tumor buds has limited clinical significance in so far as possible recurrence is concerned.

The issue of the parotid pseudocapsular form has been extensively studied as it relates to pseudocapsular vulnerability at the time of superficial parotidectomy, particularly with regard to its possible absence, microinvasion of the pseudocapsule by the tumor, tumor buds, pseudocapsular lamellation, and bosselation, defined as a smooth bulging prominence at the tumor margin. Webb and Eveson[23] retrospectively examined 126 primary pleomorphic adenomas, of which 106 were located in the parotid gland. These investigators identified an increased pseudocapsular thickness in the presence of a hypercellular tumor compared with focal pseudocapsular absence seen in hypocellular tumors (69% of cases). In addition, they found that small tumors tended to be hypercellular, whereas larger tumors (>25 mm) were hypocellular, with an inherently thinner pseudocapsule. The investigators found microinvasion of the pseudocapsule with tumor buds in 11.9% of cases. All buds were bounded by a thin fibrous pseudocapsule and were closely connected to the main tumor mass. Bosselation was noted in 76 of 126 tumors (60.3%). Exposure of the pseudocapsule was evident in 81% of the cases operated in this series. The investigators concluded that salivary gland surgeons should be prepared for precise dissection of the pseudocapsule to avoid rupture, particularly in the region of the facial nerve. Their findings indicated a frequently flimsy, variable, and uncertain border between a pleomorphic adenoma and the host tissue. They indicated that the superficial parotidectomy should guarantee at least some adequate tissue margin around the tumor.

## Partial Superficial Parotidectomy

Although the superficial parotidectomy led to a dramatic decline in local recurrence of parotid tumors when compared with the once-performed enucleation procedure, the superficial parotidectomy resulted in resection of a significant amount of normal parotid tissue, leading to a loss of parotid function. In addition, temporary facial nerve paralysis caused by complete facial nerve dissection was occasionally noted as part of the superficial parotidectomy. The observed complications of the superficial parotidectomy led many surgeons to perform a limited or partial superficial parotidectomy. This surgical procedure removes the parotid tumor surrounded by a cuff of normal parotid tissue and identifies and dissects the facial nerve only in the vicinity of the sacrifice of the parotid tumor (**Fig. 9**). Like the superficial parotidectomy, the partial superficial parotidectomy may result in an extracapsular dissection (ECD) in the vicinity of the facial nerve dissection. O'Brien[24] retrospectively evaluated 363 partial superficial parotidectomies performed on 355 patients with benign parotid disease. The incidence of immediate postoperative facial nerve weakness was 27% (98 patients), which proved to be temporary in 87 patients and permanent in 11 patients (3%). Because some of the cases

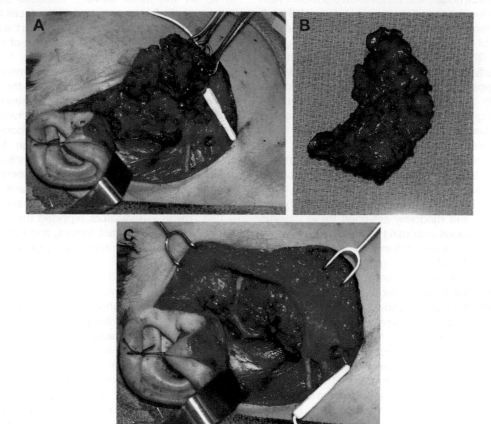

**Fig. 9.** A partial superficial parotidectomy performed for a preoperative FNAB result suggestive of pleomorphic adenoma (*A*). This surgery involved the removal of the tumor with approximately 1 cm of surrounding parotid gland (*B*). A portion of the superior and inferior aspects of the superficial lobe of the parotid gland remained at the conclusion of the partial superficial parotidectomy, and the greater auricular nerve was preserved (*C*).

operated in this series were recurrent tumors with preexisting facial nerve weakness, the incidence of permanent weakness of the facial nerve amongst the patients with intact preoperative facial nerve function was 2.5%. Three patients (0.8%) experienced recurrence of their tumors. The author indicated that partial superficial parotidectomy is the operation of choice for previously untreated localized parotid tumors lying superficial to the plane of the facial nerve. It was pointed out that most malignant tumors of the superficial lobe of the parotid gland could also be removed by this technique. Lim and colleagues[25] specifically examined the ability of the partial superficial parotidectomy to control malignant disease of the parotid gland. They retrospectively reviewed 43 patients treated with a partial superficial parotidectomy for parotid cancer confined to the superficial lobe. Sixteen tumors (37%) were high-grade and 27 tumors (63%) were low-grade. The overall survival rate and disease-free rate at 5 years were 88% and 79%, respectively. Univariate analyses showed histologic tumor grade and pathologic neck node metastases to be significant variables. Recurrences developed in 8 cases (19%); 6 of the recurrences occurred in high-grade cases and 2 of the recurrences occurred in low-grade cases. The investigators concluded by stating that partial superficial parotidectomy with appropriate postoperative radiation therapy is an oncologically acceptable procedure in the treatment of low-grade parotid cancers confined to the superficial lobe where the facial nerve is sufficiently distant from the tumor.

Roh and colleagues[26] performed a randomized clinical trial comparing partial parotidectomy versus superficial or total parotidectomy. They enrolled 101 patients with benign tumors based on FNAB and randomly assigned these patients to 1 of 2 groups according to the extent of parotidectomy: 52 underwent limited partial parotidectomy (functional surgery group) and 49 patients underwent superficial or total parotidectomy (conventional surgery group). The limited partial parotidectomy group underwent preservation of their greater auricular nerves and the main trunk of the facial nerve was identified. The overlying parotid tissue was dissected free of the nerve and maintained on the tumor with approximately 0.5 to 1.0 cm tumor-free margins. The superficial or total parotidectomy group underwent a modified Blair approach to their tumor surgery, and the greater auricular nerve was sacrificed during the surgery. A superficial or total parotidectomy was performed appropriately and all branches of the facial nerve were fully dissected. Twenty-one of 52 patients (40%) in the limited partial

parotidectomy group experienced early complications, whereas 49 of 49 (100%) patients in the superficial or total parotidectomy group experienced early complications. Temporary facial nerve weakness was noted in 23 of the 101 patients overall (22.8%) and was significantly more common in the superficial or total parotidectomy group. The fact that no tumor recurrences were noted in both groups in a 4-year follow-up period as well as other complications of less magnitude in the limited parotidectomy group justifies this approach to benign parotid tumor removal.

### Extracapsular Dissection

Extracapsular dissection (ECD) represents the most conservative and practical approach to parotid tumor surgery; a meticulous dissection immediately outside the tumor pseudocapsule is performed without intentionally identifying and dissecting the main trunk or branches of the facial nerve (**Fig. 10**). The justification of this procedure is that 60% of parotid tumors have been estimated to lie on the facial nerve.[27] Because surgical protocol calls for preservation of the facial nerve, the result is frequently a dissection along the pseudocapsule of the tumor, with no margin of normal parotid tissue in this region. It has become apparent amongst those surgeons commonly performing parotid surgery that, despite the close association of the facial nerve to the pseudocapsule of the parotid tumor, recurrence is uncommon. George and McGurk[27] reported on 156 consecutive patients with benign tumors who were operated with ECD. Complications were rare in their series, including permanent facial nerve palsy (1%), temporary facial nerve palsy (3%), sialocele (1%), and Frey's syndrome (<1%). These investigators reported that ECD is not suitable for malignant tumors, and FNAB was used routinely in the preoperative workup of their patients.

In 2003, McGurk and colleagues[28] reported on 821 patients with previously untreated epithelial parotid neoplasms in whom the preoperative diagnosis and judgment for surgery was based only on clinical examination. The tumors were classified by clinical criteria into simple tumors (clinically benign), which were discrete, mobile, and measured less than 4 cm in diameter. Complex tumors were clinically defined as those greater than 4 cm, fixed to surrounding tissues, associated with facial nerve palsy, that had deep lobe involvement, or were associated with cervical lymphadenopathy. Among the simple tumors, 503 patients underwent ECD and 159 patients underwent superficial parotidectomy. Thirty-two

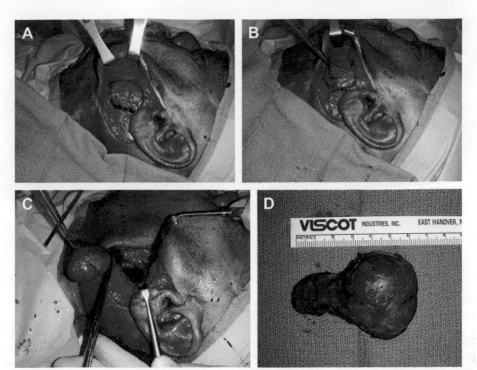

**Fig. 10.** An ECD performed for a Warthin's tumor of the left superficial lobe of the parotid gland. The proposed sacrifice of parotid tissue is marked (*A*) and the elevation of the specimen is initiated without identification of the facial nerve (*B, C*). The delivered specimen showing the handle used to assist in the retraction and procurement of the specimen (*D*). (*Images provided by* Eric Dierks, DMD, MD, FACS.)

of these 662 simple tumors (5%) proved to be carcinomas. Of these 32 patients, 12 patients underwent ECD and 20 underwent superficial parotidectomy. The 5-year and 10-year cancer-specific survival rates were 100 and 98%, respectively for ECD and superficial parotidectomy. Of the 630 patients with simple tumors and benign histologies, there were 10 recurrences at 15 years. Eight recurrences occurred after 491 ECDs (1.6%) and 2 recurrences occurred after 139 superficial parotidectomies (1.4%). The investigators concluded by stating that ECD represents a viable alternative surgical approach to superficial parotidectomy for benign tumors because there are no differences in recurrence rates as well as a reduced incidence in overall morbidity.

## Incisional Parotid Biopsy

Incisional parotid biopsy (**Fig. 11**) is rarely performed in the determination of the diagnosis of a discrete mass of the parotid gland. The primary concern with such an approach is the inherent seeding of the skin overlying the tumor such that its sacrifice is required at the time of definitive tumor surgery. In addition, the wide use of FNAB has largely replaced the need for incisional biopsy of discrete parotid masses. However, incisional parotid biopsy frequently is indicated in the

determination of the character and diagnosis of equivocal diffuse processes of the parotid gland, many of which indicate underlying systemic disease.[29] Sjögren's syndrome is perhaps the prototypical systemic disease that can be diagnosed in early stages by incisional parotid biopsy. In Marx's review[30] of 54 patients with Sjögren's syndrome, 31 (58%) had a positive labial biopsy, whereas 54 (100%) had a positive parotid biopsy. The incisional parotid biopsy also serves to rule out the presence of lymphoma in the background of Sjögren's syndrome, which is estimated to occur in approximately 5% to 10% of these patients.[7] Incisional parotid biopsy is also useful in providing an early diagnosis for otherwise equivocal cases of sarcoidosis and sialosis. Incisional biopsy of parotid neoplasms might be indicated when the tumor has eroded through the skin such that its sacrifice is already indicated at the time of surgery (**Fig. 12**). Such a biopsy is likely able to provide a more precise tissue diagnosis than FNAB.

## THE ROLE OF NECK DISSECTION IN THE MANAGEMENT OF PAROTID CANCER

The role of neck dissection in concert with superficial parotidectomy or partial superficial parotidectomy must be critically considered in the

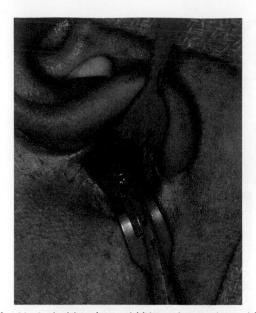

**Fig. 11.** An incisional parotid biopsy in a patient with Sjögren's syndrome that was diagnosed 10 years earlier. The recent onset of pain resulted in concern for the possibility for lymphoma such that incisional biopsy was performed. A 1-cm² specimen was procured. (*Reprinted from* Carlson ER, Ord RA, editors. Textbook and color atlas of salivary gland pathology–diagnosis and management. Ames (IA): Wiley Blackwell; 2008. p. 137; with permission.)

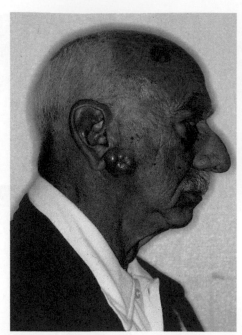

**Fig. 12.** A high-grade mucoepidermoid carcinoma of the right parotid gland, which has eroded through skin. A precise preoperative histopathologic diagnosis was offered with an incisional biopsy of the mass. A skin-sacrificing superficial parotidectomy and neck dissection were performed for this patient.

management of patients with parotid cancers. Cervical lymph node metastases have been reported to be rare in patients with cancer of the major salivary glands, with an overall incidence of clinical lymph node metastases of 16% for carcinoma of the parotid gland.[31] The thought process of the past was that elective neck dissection was seldom, if ever, indicated in the management of parotid cancer.[31,32] Moreover, it was believed that the incidence of occult nodal metastases was higher in patients with anaplastic, high-grade mucoepidermoid and salivary duct carcinoma and adenocarcinoma than in patients with low-grade mucoepidermoid and acinic cell carcinoma.[33] Other reports indicate that the overall incidence of cervical lymph node metastases from parotid cancers ranges from 18% to 28%.[34–36] Although the role of neck dissection is clear if clinically apparent lymph node metastases exist in patients with parotid cancer, a lack of consensus exists regarding the proper surgical management of the clinically negative neck. To this end, the incidence of occult cervical lymph node metastases associated with parotid cancers has been reported to be between 2% and 50%.[34,35,37,38] The observed morbidity associated with prophylactic neck dissection is insignificant. The ease of

extending the modified Blair incision inferiorly and anteriorly permits the performance of a prophylactic neck dissection in patients with parotid cancers. The realization of both issues seems to justify the near routine performance of a prophylactic neck dissection in patients with malignancies of the parotid gland. Therefore, the ability to discern malignant disease in the parotid gland is of obvious preoperative benefit, when a commitment exists to the performance of an elective neck dissection in the management of parotid cancer. The beneficial role of preoperative FNAB is clear to ablative surgeons. When the neck is treated electively, only the ipsilateral side should undergo neck dissection because contralateral lymph node metastases related to parotid cancer are negligible.[33] Armstrong and colleagues[31] indicated that a 3-level prophylactic neck dissection is statistically likely to identify occult neck disease in 90% of cases, such that a traditional supraomohyoid neck dissection is oncologically preferred.

## SUMMARY

Disease of the parotid gland is represented by a diverse array of diagnoses, ranging from acute infection to malignant neoplastic disease with facial nerve palsy. At first glance, chronic infections may resemble tumors such that the surgeon must develop an algorithm to proceed in a methodical and scientific fashion that provides early and effective treatment of patients with parotid disease. The techniques described in this discussion represent a means to that end.

## REFERENCES

1. Carlson ER. Diagnosis and management of salivary gland infections. Oral Maxillofac Surg Clin North Am 2009;21:293–312.

2. Gregoire C. Salivary gland tumors: the parotid gland. In: Bagheri S, Bell B, Ali Kahn H, editors. Current therapy in oral and maxillofacial surgery. St Louis (MO): Saunders Elsevier; 2012. p. 450–60.

3. Ellis GL, Auclair PL, Gnepp OR. Surgical pathology of the salivary glands. Philadelphia: WB Saunders; 1991.

4. Eveson JW, Cawson RA. Salivary gland tumours: a review of 2410 cases with particular reference to histological types, site, age and sex distribution. J Pathol 1985;146:51–8.

5. Spiro RH. Salivary neoplasms: overview of a 35-year experience with 2,807 patients. Head Neck Surg 1986;8:177–84.

6. Ito FA, Ito K, Vargas PA, et al. Salivary gland tumors in a Brazilian population: a retrospective study of 496 cases. Int J Oral Maxillofac Surg 2005;34:533–6.

7. Carlson ER, Ord RA. Textbook and color atlas of salivary gland pathology. Diagnosis and management. Ames (IA): Wiley Blackwell; 2008. p. 67–136.

8. Gallia LJ, Johnson JT. The incidence of neoplastic versus inflammatory disease in major salivary gland masses diagnosed by surgery. Laryngoscope 1981; 91:512–6.

9. David O, Blaney S, Hearp M. Parotid gland fine-needle aspiration cytology: an approach to differential diagnosis. Diagn Cytopathol 2007;35:47–56.

10. Zurrida S, Alasio L, Tradati N, et al. Fine-needle aspiration of parotid masses. Cancer 1993;72:2306–11.

11. Postema RJ, van Velthuysen MF, van den Brekel MWM, et al. Accuracy of fine-needle aspiration cytology of salivary gland lesions in the Netherlands Cancer Institute. Head Neck 2004;26: 418–24.

12. Atula T, Grenman R, Laippala P, et al. Fine-needle aspiration biopsy in the diagnosis of parotid gland lesions: evaluation of 438 biopsies. Diagn Cytopathol 1996;15:185–90.

13. Batsakis JG, Sneige N, El-Naggar AK. Fine needle aspiration in salivary glands: its utility and tissue effects. Ann Otol Rhinol Laryngol 1992;101:185–8.

14. Stewart CJR, MacKenzie K, McGary GW, et al. Fine-needle aspiration cytology of salivary gland: a review of 341 cases. Diagn Cytopathol 2000;22:139–46.

15. Heller KS, Dubner S, Chess Q, et al. Value of fine needle aspiration biopsy of salivary gland masses in clinical decision-making. Am J Surg 1992;164: 667–70.

16. Ali NS, Akhtar S, Junaid M, et al. Diagnostic accuracy of fine needle aspiration cytology in parotid lesions. ISRN Surg 2011;1–5. http://dx.doi.org/10.5402/2011/721525.

17. Christensen RK, Bjorndal K, Godballe C, et al. Value of fine-needle aspiration biopsy of salivary gland lesions. Head Neck 2010;32:104–8.

18. Layfield LJ. Fine-needle aspiration in the diagnosis of head and neck lesions: a review and discussion of problems in differential diagnosis. Diagn Cytopathol 2007;35:798–805.

19. Zbaren P, Guelat D, Loosli H, et al. Parotid tumors: fine-needle aspiration and/or frozen section. Otolaryngol Head Neck Surg 2008;139:811–5.

20. Bartels S, Talbot JM, DiTomasso J, et al. The relative value of fine-needle aspiration and imaging in the preoperative evaluation of parotid masses. Head Neck 2000;22:781–6.

21. Ghosh S, Panarese A, Bull PD, et al. Marginally excised parotid pleomorphic salivary adenomas: risk factors for recurrence and management. A 12.5 year mean follow-up study of histologically marginal excisions. Clin Otolaryngol Allied Sci 2003;28:262–6.

22. McGurk M, Renehan A, Gleave EN, et al. Clinical significance of the tumour capsule in the treatment of parotid pleomorphic adenomas. Br J Surg 1996; 83:1747–9.

23. Webb AJ, Eveson JW. Pleomorphic adenomas of the major salivary glands: a study of the capsular form in relation to surgical management. Clin Otolaryngol 2001;26:134–42.

24. O'Brien CJ. Current management of benign parotid tumors–the role of limited superficial parotidectomy. Head Neck 2003;25:946–52.

25. Lim YC, Lee SY, Kim K, et al. Conservative parotidectomy for the treatment of parotid cancers. Oral Oncol 2005;41:1021–7.

26. Roh JL, Kim HS, Park CI. Randomized clinical trial comparing partial parotidectomy versus superficial or total parotidectomy. Br J Surg 2007;94:1081–7.

27. George KS, McGurk M. Extracapsular dissection–minimal resection for benign parotid tumors. Br J Oral Maxillofac Surg 2011;49:451–4.

28. McGurk M, Thomas BL, Renehan AG. Extracapsular dissection for clinically benign parotid lumps: reduced morbidity without oncological compromise. Br J Cancer 2003;89:1610–3.

29. Marx RE, Hartman KS, Rethman KV. A prospective study comparing incisional labial to incisional parotid biopsies in the detection and confirmation of sarcoidosis, Sjogren's disease, sialosis and lymphoma. J Rheumatol 1988;15:621–9.

30. Marx RE. Incisional parotid biopsy for the diagnosis of systemic disease. Oral Maxillofac Surg Clin North Am 2005;7:505–17.

31. Armstrong JG, Harrison LB, Thaler HT, et al. The indications for elective treatment of the neck in cancer of the major salivary glands. Cancer 1992;69:615–9.

32. Carlson ER. Parotid tumor. In: Laskin DM, Abubaker AO, editors. Decision making in oral and maxillofacial surgery. Chicago: Quintessence; 2007. p. 212–3.

33. Medina JE. Neck dissection in the treatment of cancer of major salivary glands. Otolaryngol Clin North Am 1998;31:815–22.

34. Rodriguez-Cuevas S, Labastida L, Baena L, et al. Risk of nodal metastases from malignant salivary gland tumors related to tumor size and grade of malignancy. Eur Arch Otorhinolaryngol 1995;252: 139–42.

35. Written J, Hybert F, Hansen HS. Treatment of malignant tumors in the parotid glands. Cancer 1990;65: 2515–20.

36. Kelley D, Spiro R. Management of the neck in parotid carcinoma. Am J Surg 1996;172:695–7.

37. Gallo O, Franchi A, Bottai GV, et al. Risk factors for distant metastases from carcinoma of the parotid gland. Cancer 1996;80:844–51.

38. Santos IR, Kowalski LP, Araujo VC, et al. Multivariate analysis of risk factors for neck metastases in surgically treated parotid carcinomas. Arch Otolaryngol Head Neck Surg 2001;127:56–60.

# Robotic Surgery
## A New Approach to Tumors of the Tongue Base, Oropharynx, and Hypopharynx

Etern S. Park, DDS, MD[a], Jonathan W. Shum, DDS, MD[a],
Tuan G. Bui, MD, DMD[a,b], R. Bryan Bell, DDS, MD[a,b,c,d],
Eric J. Dierks, DMD, MD[a,b,c],*

### KEYWORDS

- Head and neck cancer • Oropharyngeal cancer • Transoral robotic surgery • Functional outcome

### KEY POINTS

- In the United States, approximately 35,000 adults will be diagnosed with squamous cell carcinoma (SCC) of the oral cavity and oropharynx every year.
- In selected patients, transoral robotic surgery (TORS) in head and neck cancer has shown acceptable surgical outcomes, with low morbidity and faster postoperative recovery.
- TORS has shown promising data to support that it provides better visualization and access to pharyngeal tumors via a minimally invasive approach, with comparable oncologic outcomes to traditional open surgery.
- TORS offers less morbidity from the operation and a better functional outcome.
- The disadvantages of TORS center on its higher costs related to purchase and maintenance of the technology.
- TORS should be prospectively compared with traditional surgical or nonsurgical options for each tumor location and stage to determine its specific role.

## INTRODUCTION

When Mr DF, a singer and bass guitar player from Oregon, first learned that he had SCC of the tonsil, he was told the cancer would require a combination of chemotherapy and radiation therapy and would probably mark the end of his singing career. If he opted for traditional surgery, his jaw and tongue would need to be split and reconstructed, leaving visible scars on his lower lip and chin. The 73-year-old musician initially agreed to undergo the recommended treatment of radiation and chemotherapy. A few days later, his surgeon called to let him know about another option—robotic surgery—which could be performed through his mouth and meant that he would not have to have his jaw and tongue divided. The musician underwent surgery on March 2010 and became one of the first patients to undergo TORS for cancer on the West Coast. Two years later, he remains cancer-free and he continues to enjoy eating, singing, and performing in his band (**Fig. 1**).

Disclosure: All authors have no financial relationships to disclose.
[a] Head and Neck Surgical Associates, 1849 Northwest Kearney, Suite 300, Portland, OR 97209; Legacy Emanuel Medical Center, 2801 North Gantenbein Avenue, Portland, OR 97227, USA; [b] Providence Portland Cancer Center, 4805 Northeast Glisan Street, Portland, OR 97213, USA; [c] Oregon Health and Science University, 611 Southwest Campus Drive, Portland, OR 97239, USA; [d] Oral, Head and Neck Cancer Program, Robert W. Franz Cancer Research Center, Providence Portland Cancer Center, 4805 Northeast Glisan Street, Portland, OR 97213, USA
* Corresponding author. Head and Neck Surgical Associates, 1849 Northwest Kearney, Suite 300, Portland, OR 97209.
E-mail address: eric.dierks@gmail.com

Oral Maxillofacial Surg Clin N Am 25 (2013) 49–59
http://dx.doi.org/10.1016/j.coms.2012.11.002
1042-3699/13/$ – see front matter © 2013 Elsevier Inc. All rights reserved.

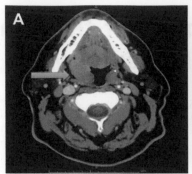
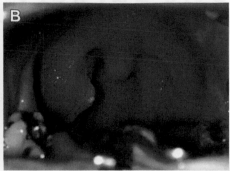

**Fig. 1.** (*A*) Right tonsillar SCC. (*arrow*) Staged as T3 tumor. (*B*) Right tonsillar SCC, appearance similar to patient DF.

Head and neck SCC affects 500,000 people worldwide per year.[1] In the United States, approximately 35,000 adults will be diagnosed with SCC of the oral cavity and oropharynx every year.[2] SCC in these sites can be treated with 1 of 3 standard treatment modalities, including surgery, radiation therapy (RT), or chemotherapy, or a combination of these. Classical oropharyngeal cancer surgery consists of en bloc resection of the tumor via lip-split mandibulotomy approach and flap reconstruction, often followed by adjuvant therapy if indicated. This treatment provided good rates of locoregional disease control. The morbidity associated with the traditional surgical approach, however, and the need to reconstruct with an insensate, adynamic flap to seal tissue planes that were widely opened for surgical access frequently resulted in incapacitating deficits in speech and swallowing. This led many physicians to prefer the use of definitive chemoradiotherapy (chemoRT) without surgery.[3,4]

The shift toward organ-sparing treatment began with the multicenter Veterans Affairs larynx study of 1991,[5] which showed that chemoRT alone could achieve cure rates equivalent to laryngectomy followed by RT while preserving the larynx. This organ-sparing philosophy, and enthusiasm for chemoRT as opposed to primary surgery, extended to other sites in the oropharynx, such as the tonsil and base of tongue. Chemotherapy plus high-dose RT (70 Gy or more) became the standard of care for oropharyngeal squamous cancer. Although concurrent chemoRT offers high rates of locoregional disease control, recent attention has been given to the significant functional deficits and diminished quality of life after intense chemoRT.

The need for head and neck cancer treatment modalities, which can offer equivalent oncologic outcomes with minimized morbidities, became the driving force to adopt a new technology. In selected patients, TORS in head and neck cancer has shown acceptable surgical outcomes with low morbidity and faster postoperative recovery. The TORS surgical defect created in the tonsillar fossa or base of tongue, although sizable, is isolated and has not been widely opened into other tissue planes. The TORS defect is simply allowed to contract and granulate, resulting in an almost fully sensate and normally dynamic healed wound. In addition to avoiding radical open surgery and the need for flap reconstruction, TORS allows better visualization of the tumor with high-definition 3-D video, which overcomes the line-of-sight limitations associated with conventional transoral laser surgery as well as improved range of motion of the surgical arms, preservation of normal adjacent structures, and shorter hospitalization.[6,7]

## MINIMALLY INVASIVE SURGERY

In the 1980s, minimally invasive surgery was introduced and rapidly spread from gynecology to general and thoracic surgery. Laparoscopic and thoracoscopic surgery offer the advantages of small incisions, reduced blood loss, shorter hospital stays, and fewer complications.[8] Limitations of the laparoscopic approach include loss of depth perception, replacement of natural hand-eye coordination with paradoxic instrument movement, and loss of dexterity. In the head and neck, the laparoscopic approach has few applications due to its limited surgical exposure and restrictions in movement of the instruments. Still, in 2003, the da Vinci (Intuitive Surgical, Sunnyvale, CA) system was first described as a means of minimizing incisions in the neck.[9]

## HISTORY OF ROBOTIC SURGERY

Leonardo da Vinci, the Renaissance painter and scientist, is credited for designing and building the robot in human form around in the year 1495.[10] It was not until the mid-twentieth century that his sketches and diagrams were recognized as prototypes for modern robots. It is fitting that the most widely used Food and Drug Administration (FDA)-approved surgical robot in today is named, *da Vinci*.

Although robots have been used in industries, such as automobile manufacturing, for decades, the first surgical robot was the Programmable Universal Machine for Assembly (PUMA), which was used for stereotactic brain biopsies and for resection of an astrocytoma of the thalamus in 1985.[11,12] The United States military and the National Aeronautics and Space Administration recognized the concept of telepresence surgery, which entails the possibility of having a highly skilled surgeon available to the battlefront from a safe, remote site to perform surgery on wounded soldiers. Although telepresence surgery never found application in the military, their efforts accelerated the development of robots in medical applications today.

In 1992, the ROBODOC (Curexo Technology Corporation, Fremont, CA) was introduced in orthopedic surgery. Its role as a robot was limited to milling of the femoral cavity for hip replacement surgery.[13] A year later, Wang developed the Automated Endoscopic System for Optimal Positioning (AESOP), which was used in laparoscopic surgery to enable surgeons to control the robotic arm and video laparoscope either manually or with a surgeon's voice.[14] In 1999, the ZEUS system, consisting of 3 robotic arms and a voice-controlled endoscope holder arm, was used by Reichenspurnen and colleagues[15] for performing 2 aortocoronary bypasses. The limitations of rigid equipment and a 2-D view of the surgical field without depth perception led to development of the current da Vinci Surgical System by Intuitive Surgical.[16,17] The first da Vinci surgical robot head and neck operation that was successfully performed on a human was the excision of vallecular cyst.[18]

## THE DA VINCI SYSTEM

Although robots have been described in science fiction as autonomous and preprogrammed machines, the surgical robot is neither. Conceptually, it is an extension of a surgeon's hands and mind to the surgical field. The da Vinci system is the primary robotic system in use today in the field of medicine.[19] It consists of 3 major components, each of which is independently mobile:

1. The surgeon console: The surgeon is immersed in high-definition video in 3-D for true perception of depth, allowing a virtual extension of the surgeon's hands into a patient's body. The surgeon's thumb and third finger engage

the hand units that control the instruments and that scale down movement to 5:1. A filtration module eliminates hand tremor. Pedals are used for cautery, for camera movement, and to clutch for optimal position of the instruments.

2. The robotic cart: This allows the surgeon to manipulate up to 3 EndoWrist (Intuitive Surgical, Sunnyvale, California) instruments, although only 2 are used for TORS. EndoWrist instruments provide 7° of freedom and 90° of articulation as well as tremor reduction (**Fig. 2**). The robotic telescope contains 2 cameras in the distal tip, which are separated by 15°. Each camera transmits an image to a different eye, allowing a truly stereoscopic view of the surgical field (**Fig. 3**).

3. The vision cart: This contains the light source and the dual camera and supports the monitor, which displays a high-definition image of the surgical field to a bedside assistant, other members of the surgical team, and observers.[17]

The surgeon is not scrubbed and is seated at the operating console. The bedside assistant is scrubbed and is seated at the patient's head and assists with suction and retraction. The scrub nurse and instrument table are located by the patient on the opposite side of the bedside assistant, allowing efficient communication among surgical team members and minimizing obstruction (**Fig. 4**).

For a TORS case, the patient is intubated orally with a reinforced endotracheal tube, which is sutured to the contralateral buccal mucosa. The patient is rotated 180° away from the anesthesiologist. The patient's eyes are protected using an

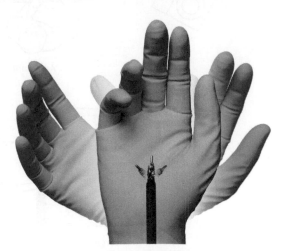

**Fig. 2.** Hand instrument articulation showing range of motion. (Copyright © 2012, Intuitive Surgical.)

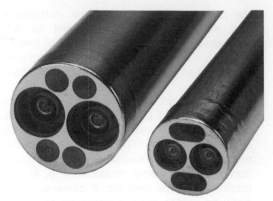

**Fig. 3.** 12 mm and 8.5 mm Endoscope. Two lenses allow stereoscopic view of the surgical field. (Copyright © 2012, Intuitive Surgical.)

adhesive plastic eye shield, and the maxillary teeth are often protected with dental guard. Either the McIvor retractor or the Feyh-Kastenbauer-Weinstein-O'Malley retractor is placed and rigidly

secured to the operating table for optimal surgical exposure and visualization. Proper placement and fixation of the retractor are critical for success in TORS. The robot is docked at a 30° angle to the operating table. The camera arm is then positioned centrally, and arms 1 and 2 are positioned on either side of the camera arm, allowing optimal range of movement with minimal collisions. Arm 3 is not used in TORS and it is positioned out of the way (**Fig. 5**).

## TORS INDICATIONS FOR HEAD AND NECK CANCER

Tonsil and base of the tongue resections are the most commonly performed procedures with TORS.

Indications for TORS for oropharyngeal cancer are[19]

1. The tumor must be adequately visualized and exposed for resection. Consider characteristics,

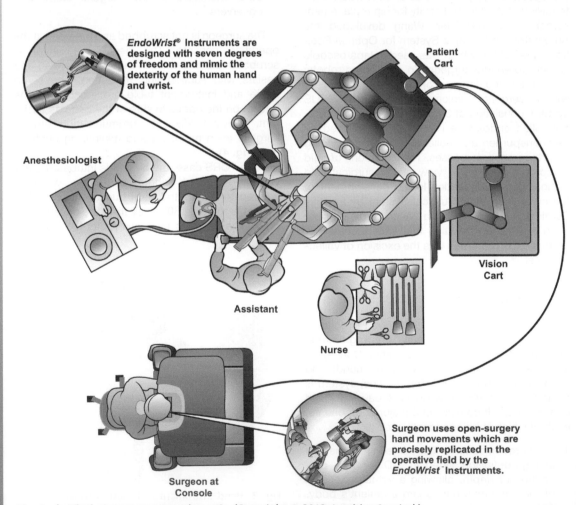

*EndoWrist®* Instruments are designed with seven degrees of freedom and mimic the dexterity of the human hand and wrist.

Patient Cart

Anesthesiologist

Vision Cart

Assistant

Nurse

Surgeon uses open-surgery hand movements which are precisely replicated in the operative field by the *EndoWrist™* Instruments.

Surgeon at Console

**Fig. 4.** da Vinci operating room schematic. (Copyright © 2012, Intuitive Surgical.)

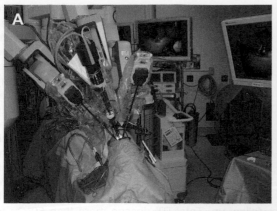
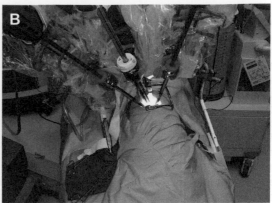
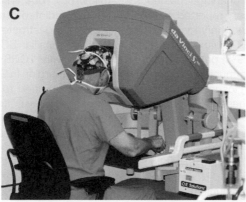

**Fig. 5.** (*A*) TORS set up. (*B*) TORS set up, close-up. (*C*) Surgeon operating from da Vinci console.

such as trismus, anteriorly positioned larynx, macroglossia, and morbid obesity, which may make retractor placement difficult.

2. The tumor must be amenable to negative margin resection with TORS.

Contraindications for oropharyngeal TORS include[20]

1. Tumor invading the mandible
2. Unresectability of involved neck nodes
3. Resection requiring more that 50% of the tongue base
4. Resection requiring more than 50% of the posterior pharyngeal wall
5. Radiologic confirmation of carotid artery involvement
6. Prevertebral fascia fixation of the tumor

Neck dissection may be performed concurrently or in a delayed fashion. Postoperatively, a decision is made whether to keep the patient intubated due to edema. In the authors' institution, most patients who undergo base of tongue resection remain intubated overnight, and most who undergo radical tonsillectomy are extubated in the operating room after surgery.

## CONCURRENT NECK DISSECTION WITH TORS

With TORS, many surgeons have avoided concurrent neck dissection, and staging of the neck dissection was preferred to avoid creating a pharyngocutaneous communication and to avoid bathing the exposed carotid artery in saliva. The addition of laryngopharyngeal swelling from concurrent neck dissection may necessitate tracheostomy.[20] Staged neck dissection after primary tumor resection can provide additional benefits, including decreased need for tracheostomy and allowing the surgeon to readdress the primary tumor site at the time of neck dissection if the final surgical margins are positive for malignancy. Staging the neck also helps to maximize the usage of the da Vinci robot by other surgeons by decreasing the operating time of a TORS case in the robot room in a high volume institution.[21] Weinstein and colleagues[20] demonstrated acceptable outcomes with TORS radical tonsillectomy in 27 patients and advocated staged neck dissection in 1 to 3 weeks. Their rationale for staged neck dissection was to avoid a connection between the pharynx and the neck and to minimize neck swelling.

Staged neck dissection, however, carries an inherent financial burden and risks. It contributes to increased overall treatment cost due to multiple hospitalizations and it potentially delays recommended adjuvant therapy. Ang and colleagues[22] and Peteras and Withers[23] demonstrated a greater than 6-week interval between initial surgery, and postoperative RT yielded significantly lower locoregional control rates in patients receiving the 7-week scheduled RT. They recommended completion of the RT in a cumulative time of less than 13 weeks from the ablative surgery. Holsinger and colleagues[24] reported 191 oropharyngectomies with simultaneous neck dissection. None of these patients developed pharyngocutaneous fistula. Moore and colleagues[21] reported on 148 consecutive patients with oropharyngeal carcinoma who underwent TORS with concurrent neck dissection. Forty-two (29%) patients had intraoperative orocervical communication, which was repaired with primary closure or pedicled locoregional muscle flap. Of these, 6 (4%) patients were managed with outpatient incision and drainage with packing. In the authors' institution, 25 patients have undergone TORS for oropharyngeal carcinoma to date. Ten (40%) patients had simultaneous neck dissection. None of these patients had orocervical communication or required tracheotomy. TORS with concurrent neck dissection can be performed safely in many patients without delaying adjuvant therapy or compromising safety.

## TORS AND QUALITY OF LIFE

Tumor control and survival rate are considered the most important measures of treatment efficacy for patients with primary oropharyngeal SCC. Studies using aggressive and uncompromised RT with concurrent chemotherapy have consistently demonstrated a survival and locoregional disease control benefit.[25,26] This benefit, however, has not come without drawbacks. Levendag and colleagues[27] demonstrated a steep dose-effect relationship, with an increase of the probability of dysphasia of 19% with every additional 10 Gy after 55 Gy in RT. In addition to dysphasia, the adverse effects associated with RT are well known to oral and maxillofacial surgeons and include trismus, osteoradionecrosis, xerostomia, and radiation dental caries.[28,29]

In multiple studies, TORS demonstrated favorable surgical as well as functional outcomes. Weinstein and colleagues[30] reported a 100% regional disease control rate after TORS and selective neck dissection for oropharyngeal carcinoma in 31 patients; 71% of those patients received RT or combined chemoRT. None of patients required permanent gastrostomy, and all patients were tolerating oral intake at 2-year follow-up. TORS has the potential to avoid the lower total health-related quality of life that has been independently associated with gastrostomy and history of RT among head and neck cancer patients.[31] Li and colleagues,[32] at the University of California, Davis, Comprehensive Cancer Center, reported that when head and neck cancers were treated by definitive concurrent chemotherapy and intensity-modulated radiation therapy without surgery, 44% of patients were gastrostomy tube-dependent at their 6-month follow-up. Total RT dosage more than 60 Gy to 62 Gy predicted greater than 50% probability of prolonged gastrostomy dependence. By comparison, 27 tonsillar SCC patients were successfully treated with TORS by obtaining negative final surgical margins in 93% of patients; 96% of these patients returned to oral intake without the need for gastrostomy.[20] If oropharyngeal cancer treated with TORS results in negative margins and if none of the cervical nodes harbor metastases, postoperative RT is unnecessary. If postoperative RT is indicated after TORS surgery because of positive margins or greater than one positive cervical node, it is feasible to reduce the dose of postoperative RT, often without concurrent chemotherapy. Deintensified radiotherapy to the primary tumor site with selective doses to higher risk areas of the neck limits deterioration of swallowing function.[30] TORS provides a function-preserving alternative treatment of oropharyngeal tumors. With less gastrostomy dependence, reduced need for tracheostomy, and less surgical morbidity, TORS provides favorable functional outcomes.

## COST EFFECTIVENESS

The cost of medical care increases as technologic innovation in diagnosis and treatment develops. A new technology can become accepted as a standard of care if it improves survival rate or quality of life. If a new technology cannot improve surgical outcomes, it must demonstrate reduction in the cost of treatment to justify use of the new technology. Does TORS demonstrate an improved survival rate and quality of life to justify the increase in the cost of use of the robot?

Robotic surgical system use has rapidly increased in the past few years. By 2007, approximately 800 da Vinci robots were installed in US hospitals. As of March 2012, 1615 units were performing 360,000 procedures yearly.[33] The costs of operation are primarily determined by equipment cost, duration of operation, and length of hospitalization.[34] Initial costs of TORS include the da Vinci Surgical System ($1–$2.3 million), an annual service contract ($100,000–$170,000/year), and instruments ($2000/instrument, each of which may be used for only 10 cases).[17] If 300 cases are performed annually, the robot adds approximately $1000 per case over 7 years to cover initial da Vinci robot acquisition cost.[35]

Operating room costs are significantly different among hospitals. A study of 100 US hospitals showed that operating room charges averaged $62 per minute (range $21.80–$133.12).[36] Hillel and colleagues[37] pointed out increased total operative time due to operating room setup as potentially limiting routine use of the da Vinci robot. McLeod and Melder[18] reported the first use of da Vinci robot in laryngeal surgery in 2005. A vallecular cyst was excised without complication and the patient was discharged the same day. The total operative time was 109 minutes, 89 minutes of which was spent setting up the robot. A significant decrease in the robot setup time has been reported as experience with TORS increases.[38] In a series of 150 patients with oral cavity or laryngopharyngeal lesions in a high-volume institution, an average additional setup time to achieve exposure and robotic positioning for TORS was 4 minutes when compared with the exposure time for standard transoral resection.[39] Considering the costs of increased operative time with setting up robot and equipment, the additional cost for TORS with an experienced operator is approximately $1300 per case ($1000 for robotic equipment and $300 for increased operating room time cost per case).[35,36]

The main factor contributing to the higher cost per case is the initial cost of purchasing the robot. The addition of a trained TORS surgeon can create a TORS program at an institution that already has a robot that was purchased for other high-volume uses (ie, cardiac, gynecologic, or urological procedures). The addition of TORS cases adds to the value of the robot already purchased by the institution.[40] Intuitive Surgical is the only manufacturer of a surgical robot at this time, and the cost of robotic operation may decline if there is more competition in the surgical robot market in the future.[41] Long-term prospective oncologic outcome studies and direct cost analysis comparing TORS with other treatment modalities must be conducted for TORS to assert itself as the standard of care for selected head and neck cancer treatment.

## RISKS/LIMITATIONS

Since Mohr and colleagues[42] performed the first mitral valve repairs by using an early prototype of the da Vinci system in 1998, the da Vinci system has established a strong record of overall device safety. A multicenter trial at 10 US institutions showed 112 mitral valve repairs were performed with da Vinci robots safely and without intraoperative conversions to alternative surgical techniques (eg, sternotomy or thoracotomy enlargement).[43] Has a comparable safety record has been observed in TORS?

Surgeons may have difficulty in transitioning from a wide-access, direct vision head and neck operation to telemanipulation of tissue in restricted spaces because of the potential limitation in the control of bleeding in oropharyngeal and laryngeal surgery. In TORS, the excellent visualization of surgical field and the use of monopolar and bipolar cautery instruments aid the maintenance of hemostasis. Robotic radical prostatectomy has been performed in large series of patients with low morbidity and significantly less operative blood loss than standard retropubic prostatectomy.[44] Hockstein and colleagues[45] conducted canine robotic surgery for evaluation of the ability to control bleeding in TORS. Both large and small vessel hemostasis was obtained with robot-controlled monopolar and bipolar cautery and small hemoclips. Large hemoclips were applied by a bedside assistant surgeon for management of large arterial vessels. Effective hemostasis can be obtained with control of both large and small vessels using hemoclips and electrocautery in TORS, and any bleeding from mucosa or muscle edges is essentially eliminated with the use of both monopolar and bipolar cautery. Excellent visualization of the surgical field through 3-D optics allows easy identification of vessels, aiding effective hemostasis with electrocautery and hemoclips.

The FDA maintains a Manufacturer and User Facility Device Experience (MAUDE) database, which documents reports of adverse events involving medical devices. Since inception of the da Vinci robot, 63 deaths associated with it have been reported. None of the deaths, however, was caused by the da Vinci surgical system. Of 63, 6 mortalities were associated with TORS, consisting of 3 patients with postoperative hemorrhage after base of tongue resection, 2 patients with pulmonary infection after partial laryngectomy, and 1 patient with unknown cause.[46]

The University of Pennsylvania Head and Neck Surgery group simulated potential complications related to device misuse or malfunction by intentionally injuring human cadavers by gross robot device misuse.[47] The simulation demonstrated that intact teeth could not be fractured and that forcefully impaling the skin and mucosa with robotic instruments resulted only in superficial lacerations. The cervical spine or mandible could not be fractured. Orbits may potentially be injured by the robotic instruments; however, the safety goggles could not be broken by intentionally traumatizing them with the robotic endoscope and instruments. It seems that use of the surgical robot does not add substantial risk to transoral surgery.

## TRAINING SURGEONS AND TORS PROGRAM IMPLEMENTATION

Introducing a new and complex technology to an institution involves many challenges. Resistance to change may come from hospital administration or operating room support staff or within surgical services themselves. Since the approval of the da Vinci robot for use in TORS by the FDA in December 2009, there have been no concrete guidelines to assist the introduction of a TORS program to an institution.[38] The steps required for adaptation of any new technology include an assessment of the evidence-based efficacy of the procedure, provision of methodical education for surgeons to acquire knowledge and skills, intraoperative safety monitoring, credentialing and privileging of surgeons, and education of patients.[48]

Richmon and colleagues[38] at Johns Hopkins Hospital showed that a TORS program can be implemented efficiently and safely following a stepwise approach. Surgeons must attend a TORS course involving animal surgery provided by Intuitive Surgical and must complete an online program. This is followed by performing robotic procedures on cadavers and observation of live and video TORS procedures at 1 of 17 da Vinci Robot training centers in the United States. On returning to the surgeon's institution, the surgeon prepares the TORS team by defining the team leader and dedicated bedside assistant with robotic training and establishes emergency plans in case of uncontrolled bleeding, airway compromise, or robot malfunction. A mock surgical case using a full-body mannequin can be simulated with a team consisting of a robotic surgeon, nurses, and anesthesiologist. Depending on the hospital protocol, initial live surgical procedures may be proctored by an experienced TORS-certified surgeon. Early experience at Johns Hopkins, with their first 20 TORS cases, showed an average positioning time of 38 ± 13 minutes, which includes patient positioning, direct laryngoscopy, and robot docking. They found no significant difference in setup time between the first 10 cases and the second 10 cases, which is in contrast to other reports, which demonstrated a steep learning

curve with the initial setup.[6,49] Richmon and colleagues[38] and Lawson and colleagues[50] credited a mock TORS-simulated case with a mannequin with providing an opportunity to address the details and complexities of room setup and positioning. Negative surgical margins were obtained in all 20 cases and average hospitalization time was 1.3 days. All patients were discharged on an oral diet. With stepwise preparation for the TORS program, favorable outcomes and efficiency can be achieved on program initiation.

Besides the efforts of the entire TORS team to run cases efficiently without compromising patient safety, the surgeon's learning curve must be addressed. When a surgeon is learning a new surgical technique, inherent limitations are present that may result in outcomes inferior to what might otherwise have been obtained with an experienced surgeon. It has been reported that a surgeon must perform between 8 to 12 and as many as 200 cases to become proficient in a urological procedure with the da Vinci robot.[51] Currently no data are available to estimate how many TORS cases a surgeon must perform to become proficient. Intuitive Surgical has introduced a surgical simulator for the da Vinci robot, but its exercises are not geared to TORS practice. Standardized competency evaluation paired with long-term oncological outcome is warranted.

## TRAINING RESIDENTS

Ethical, economic, and legal concerns must be addressed within the context of the acquisition of new technical surgical skills in resident training.[52] In 1995, the American College of Surgeons published a statement on 4 issues to be considered before a new surgical technology is applied to the care of patients: (1) Has it been adequately tested for safety and efficacy? (2) Is it at least as safe and effective as existing, proved techniques? (3) Is the surgeon fully qualified to use it? and (4) Is it cost effective?[53] Present data support the concept that TORS can be performed safely and effectively and arguably cost-effectively. It was not until 2009 that robotic assistance became an important treatment modality for head and neck surgery. Most, if not all, of current TORS training programs are geared toward the training of attending surgeons. Unlike other surgical subspecialties, including urology, gynecology, colorectal surgery, general surgery, and cardiothoracic surgery, no training standards or competency verification has been set for the TORS surgical trainee.[54]

Most robotic training occurs during live surgery or robotic courses on animal models. Training with an animal model may provide familiarization with the surgical console, but it lacks the specific technical aspects of a procedure on a human patient. Training during live surgery may expose patients to the inherent risks associated with an inexperienced surgeon.[55] Lerner and colleagues[55] demonstrated that training with a virtual reality robotic simulator group had a similar significant improvement in both timing and accuracy score when compared with the group who only had training with the da Vinci surgical robot. The use of a virtual simulator may help surgical residents to acquire robotic skill safely before performing live robot-assisted surgery in a low-volume institution. TORS is inherently low volume and comprises a small portion of the total number of robot-assisted surgeries performed, which in turn limits the opportunity for resident TORS training. In the presence of low TORS case volume and with limited training opportunities at a TORS training center for residents, the robotic simulator can be a valuable training tool in the field of head and neck surgery.

Traditionally, the qualification to perform a procedure has been determined by the number of cases completed during training. Currently, however, there is no supporting evidence that performing a certain number of cases leads to performance of safe and efficient robotic surgery. A standardized assessment tool to measure robotic surgical skills—the Global Evaluative Assessment of Robotic Skills (GEARS)—has been developed by Goh and colleagues[54] at Baylor College of Medicine. This showed excellent consistency, reliability, and validity in evaluating trainees' robotic surgical expertise. GEARS is composed of 6 domains: depth perception, bimanual dexterity, efficiency, force sensitivity, autonomy, and robotic control. Even though GEARS was developed based on urological robotic procedures, evaluation criteria were not operation specific. It seems that GEARS may be useful to assess progression in resident TORS training.

Another useful tool for robotic surgery teaching is an integrated dual-console station.[19] With a dual-console da Vinci robot, a student can perform the surgery while an attending surgeon can direct movement with visible pointers or can take over control of the robotic arms from a separate surgical console.

## FUTURE APPLICATIONS/TELESURGERY

All current robotic surgeries are performed by a surgeon in the same operating room as the patient. In telesurgery, the surgeon operates at a significant distance from the patient. The first human long-distance operation with a robot was successfully performed by Marescaux and colleageus,[56] who performed a cholecystectomy in which the surgeon was in New York and the patient in Paris. As with the military application of telepresence surgery, telesurgery may offer timely access for surgical treatment, especially for emergency operations in the setting of a scientific mission in a remote area or in a small rural hospital where surgeons are not readily available.

## SUMMARY

Head and neck SCC is primarily treated with surgery or definitive chemoRT and both have shown similar locoregional disease control and overall survival. TORS has shown promising data to support that it provides better visualization and access to pharyngeal tumors via a minimally invasive approach, with comparable oncologic outcomes to traditional open surgery. More importantly, TORS offers less morbidity from the operation and a better functional outcome. The disadvantages of TORS center on its higher costs related to purchase and maintenance of the technology. Encouraging results of robotic surgery are reported, but definitive indications are yet to be determined. TORS should be prospectively compared with traditional surgical or nonsurgical options for each tumor location and stage to determine its specific role.

## REFERENCES

1. Parkin DM, Bray F, Ferlay J, et al. Estimating the world cancer burden: Globocan 2000. Int J Cancer 2001;94(2):153–6.
2. American Cancer Society. Available at: http://www.cancer.org/Cancer/OralCavityandOropharyngealCancer/DetailedGuide/oral-cavity-and-oropharyngeal-cancer-key-statistics. Accessed May 5, 2012.
3. Chen AY, Schrag N, Hao Y, et al. Changes in treatment of advanced laryngeal cancer 1985-2001. Otolaryngol Head Neck Surg 2006;135(6):831–7.
4. Chen AY, Schrag N, Hao Y, et al. Changes in treatment of advanced oropharyngeal cancer, 1985-2001. Laryngoscope 2007;117(1):16–21.
5. The Department of Veterans Affairs Laryngeal Cancer Study Group. Induction chemotherapy plus radiation compared with surgery plus radiation in patients with advanced laryngeal cancer. N Engl J Med 1991;324(24):1685–90.
6. Moore EJ, Olsen KD, Kasperbauer JL. Transoral robotic surgery for oropharyngeal squamous cell carcinoma: a prospective study of feasibility and functional outcomes. Laryngoscope 2009;119(11):2156–64.

7. O'Malley BW Jr, Weinstein GS, Snyder W, et al. Transoral robotic surgery (TORS) for base of tongue neoplasms. Laryngoscope 2006;116(8):1465–72.

8. Holsinger FC, Sweeney AD, Jantharapattana K, et al. The emergence of endoscopic head and neck surgery. Curr Oncol Rep 2010;12(3):216–22.

9. Gourin CG, Terris DJ. Surgical robotics in otolaryngology: expanding the technology envelope. Curr Opin Otolaryngol Head Neck Surg 2004;12(3):204–8.

10. Rosheim M. Leonardo's lost robots. Heidelberg (Germany): Springer; 2006. p. 69.

11. Drake JM, Joy M, Goldenberg A, et al. Computer- and robot-assisted resection of thalamic astrocytomas in children. Neurosurgery 1991;29(1):27–33.

12. Kwoh YS, Hou J, Jonckheere EA, et al. A robot with improved absolute positioning accuracy for CT guided stereotactic brain surgery. IEEE Trans Biomed Eng 1988;35(2):153–60.

13. Cowley G. Introducing "Robodoc". A robot finds his calling—in the operating room. Newsweek 1992; 120(21):86.

14. Sackier JM, Wang Y. Robotically assisted laparasopic surgery. From concept to development. Surg Endosc 1994;8(1):63–6.

15. Reichenspurner H, Damiano RJ, Mack M, et al. Use of the voice-controlled and computer-assisted surgical system ZEUS for endoscopic coronary artery bypass grafting. J Thorac Cardiovasc Surg 1999;118(1):11–6.

16. Nguyen NT, Hinojosa MW, Finley D, et al. Application of robotics in general surgery: initial experience. Am Surg 2004;70(10):914–7.

17. Available at: http://www.intuitivesurgical.com/company/history/system.html. Accessed May 15, 2012.

18. McLeod IK, Melder PC. Da Vinci robot-assisted excision of a vallecular cyst: a case report. Ear Nose Throat J 2005;84(3):170–2.

19. Newman JG, Kuppersmith RB, O'Malley BW Jr. Robotics and telesurgery in otolaryngology. Otolaryngol Clin North Am 2011;44(6):1317–31, viii.

20. Weinstein GS, O'Malley BW Jr, Snyder W, et al. Transoral robotic surgery: radical tonsillectomy. Arch Otolaryngol Head Neck Surg 2007;133(12):1220–6.

21. Moore EJ, Olsen KD, Martin EJ. Concurrent neck dissection and transoral robotic surgery. Laryngoscope 2011;121(3):541–4.

22. Ang KK, Trotti A, Brown BW, et al. Randomized trial addressing risk features and time factors of surgery plus radiotherapy in advanced head-and-neck cancer. Int J Radiat Oncol Biol Phys 2001;51(3):571–8.

23. Peters LJ, Withers HR. Applying radiobiological principles to combined modality treatment of head and neck cancer–the time factor. Int J Radiat Oncol Biol Phys 1997;39(4):831–6.

24. Holsinger FC, McWhorter AJ, Menard M, et al. Transoral lateral oropharyngectomy for squamous cell carcinoma of the tonsillar region: I. Technique, complications, and functional results. Arch Otolaryngol Head Neck Surg 2005;131(7):583–91.

25. Adelstein DJ, Saxton JP, Lavertu P, et al. A phase III randomized trial comparing concurrent chemotherapy and radiotherapy with radiotherapy alone in resectable stage III and IV squamous cell head and neck cancer: preliminary results. Head Neck 1997;19(7):567–75.

26. Wendt TG, Grabenbauer GG, Rodel CM, et al. Simultaneous radiochemotherapy versus radiotherapy alone in advanced head and neck cancer: a randomized multicenter study. J Clin Oncol 1998; 16(4):1318–24.

27. Levendag PC, Teguh DN, Voet P, et al. Dysphagia disorders in patients with cancer of the oropharynx are significantly affected by the radiation therapy dose to the superior and middle constrictor muscle: a dose-effect relationship. Radiother Oncol 2007; 85(1):64–73.

28. Lee WR, Mendenhall WM, Parsons JT, et al. Carcinoma of the tonsillar region: a multivariate analysis of 243 patients treated with radical radiotherapy. Head Neck 1993;15(4):283–8.

29. Fein DA, Lee WR, Amos WR, et al. Oropharyngeal carcinoma treated with radiotherapy: a 30-year experience. Int J Radiat Oncol Biol Phys 1996; 34(2):289–96.

30. Weinstein GS, Quon H, O'Malley BW Jr, et al. Selective neck dissection and deintensified postoperative radiation and chemotherapy for oropharyngeal cancer: a subset analysis of the University of Pennsylvania transoral robotic surgery trial. Laryngoscope 2010;120(9):1749–55.

31. Rogers LQ, Rao K, Malone J, et al. Factors associated with quality of life in outpatients with head and neck cancer 6 months after diagnosis. Head Neck 2009;31(9):1207–14.

32. Li B, Li D, Lau DH, et al. Clinical-dosimetric analysis of measures of dysphagia including gastrostomy-tube dependence among head and neck cancer patients treated definitively by intensity-modulated radiotherapy with concurrent chemotherapy. Radiat Oncol 2009;4:52.

33. Available at: http://investor.intuitivesurgical.com/phoenix.zhtml?c=122359&p=irol-IRHome. Accessed May 15, 2012.

34. Lotan Y. Is robotic surgery cost-effective: no. Curr Opin Urol 2012;22(1):66–9.

35. Bolenz C, Gupta A, Hotze T, et al. Cost comparison of robotic, laparoscopic, and open radical prostatectomy for prostate cancer. Eur Urol 2010;57(3):453–8.

36. Shippert RD. A study of time-dependent operating room fees and how to save $100000 by using time-saving products. Am J Cosmetic Surg 2005; 22(1):25–34.

37. Hillel AT, Kapoor A, Simaan N, et al. Applications of robotics for laryngeal surgery. Otolaryngol Clin North Am 2008;41(4):781–91, vii.

38. Richmon JD, Agrawal N, Pattani KM. Implementation of a TORS program in an academic medical center. Laryngoscope 2011;121(11):2344–8.

39. Weinstein GS, O'Malley BW Jr, Snyder W, et al. Transoral robotic surgery: supraglottic partial laryngectomy. Ann Otol Rhinol Laryngol 2007;116(1):19–23.

40. Weinstein GS, O'Malley BW Jr, Desai SC, et al. Transoral robotic surgery: does the ends justify the means? Curr Opin Otolaryngol Head Neck Surg 2009;17(2):126–31.

41. Barbash GI, Glied SA. New technology and health care costs—the case of robot-assisted surgery. N Engl J Med 2010;363(8):701–4.

42. Mohr FW, Falk V, Diegeler A, et al. Minimally invasive port-access mitral valve surgery. J Thorac Cardiovasc Surg 1998;115(3):567–74 [discussion: 574–66].

43. Nifong LW, Chitwood WR, Pappas PS, et al. Robotic mitral valve surgery: a United States multicenter trial. J Thorac Cardiovasc Surg 2005;129(6):1395–404.

44. Parsons JK, Bennett JL. Outcomes of retropubic, laparoscopic, and robotic-assisted prostatectomy. Urology 2008;72(2):412–6.

45. Hockstein NG, Weinstein GS, O'Malley BW Jr. Maintenance of hemostasis in transoral robotic surgery. ORL J Otorhinolaryngol Relat Spec 2005;67(4):220–4.

46. Available at: www.accessdata.fda.gov/scripts/cdrh/cfdocs/cfMAUDE/search.cfm. Accessed May 12, 2012.

47. Hockstein NG, O'Malley BW Jr, Weinstein GS. Assessment of intraoperative safety in transoral robotic surgery. Laryngoscope 2006;116(2):165–8.

48. Sachdeva AK, Russell TR. Safe introduction of new procedures and emerging technologies in surgery: education, credentialing, and privileging. Surg Oncol Clin N Am 2007;16(1):101–14.

49. Genden EM, Desai S, Sung CK. Transoral robotic surgery for the management of head and neck cancer: a preliminary experience. Head Neck 2009;31(3):283–9.

50. Lawson G, Matar N, Remacle M, et al. Transoral robotic surgery for the management of head and neck tumors: learning curve. Eur Arch Otorhinolaryngol 2011;268(12):1795–801.

51. Frota R, Turna B, Barros R, et al. Comparison of radical prostatectomy techniques: open, laparoscopic and robotic assisted. Int Braz J Urol 2008;34(3):259–68 [discussion: 268–9].

52. Bridges M, Diamond DL. The financial impact of teaching surgical residents in the operating room. Am J Surg 1999;177(1):28–32.

53. Statement on issues to be considered before new surgical technology is applied to the care of patients. Committee on Emerging Surgical Technology and Education of American College of Surgeons. Bull Am Coll Surg 1995;80:46–7.

54. Goh AC, Goldfarb DW, Sander JC, et al. Global evaluative assessment of robotic skills: validation of a clinical assessment tool to measure robotic surgical skills. J Urol 2012;187(1):247–52.

55. Lerner MA, Ayalew M, Peine WJ, et al. Does training on a virtual reality robotic simulator improve performance on the da Vinci surgical system? J Endourol 2010;24(3):467–72.

56. Marescaux J, Leroy J, Rubino F, et al. Transcontinental robot-assisted remote telesurgery: feasibility and potential applications. Ann Surg 2002;235(4):487–92.

# Fluorescence Angiography in the Assessment of Flap Perfusion and Vitality

Melvyn S. Yeoh, DMD, MD, D. David Kim, DMD, MD*,
G.E. Ghali, DDS, MD

## KEYWORDS

- Fluorescence angiography • Pedicle flap • Reconstruction • Free-tissue transfer

## KEY POINTS

- Intraoperative Fluorescence angiography is increasingly being adopted by reconstructive surgeons for use in pedicled tissue flaps and microvascular free-tissue transfer procedures.
- The ease of use and the need for minimal amounts of equipment make it advantageous for surgical teams to use intraoperatively.
- At present, the main disadvantage of this technology is its cost; but with time and greater adoption of this technology, the cost will eventually decrease.
- Decreased postoperative complications and reduced need for revision surgery with the use of this technology will play a significant role in decreasing the overall health care costs for these complex reconstructive procedures.

 Videos of fluorescence angiography accompany this article at http://www.oralmaxsurgery. theclinics.com/

## INTRODUCTION

Pedicled flaps and free-tissue transfers have become invaluable tools for reconstruction of the head and neck region. These methods are used routinely to reconstruct hard and soft tissue defects, but compromised blood supply and subsequent flap failure remains a constant concern for the surgeon, particularly in free-tissue transfer. Early detection of vascular compromise and its prompt correction are thus critical to the success of these procedures.

Many intraoperative and postoperative monitoring devices have been developed to help prevent and identify vessel occlusion, with varying degrees of success. At present, the gold standard in evaluation of microvascular reconstruction remains clinical evaluation of color, turgor, bleeding, and warmth of the exposed soft tissue paddle.[1] Several noninvasive and invasive technologies have been developed to enhance the accuracy of the clinical examination, but none of these devices has been universally adopted. Noninvasive techniques include hand-held Doppler ultrasound, infrared thermography, polarized spectral imaging, and laser Doppler perfusion imaging. Invasive techniques include implantable Doppler probes, microdialysis, and venous pressure measurements with

Funding: No funding was received or solicited for this article.

Conflict of interest: Dr Kim is a consultant for LifeCell Corporation.

Department of Oral and Maxillofacial/Head and Neck Surgery, Louisiana State University Health Science Center Shreveport, 1501 Kings Highway, PO Box 33932, Shreveport, LA 71130, USA

* Corresponding author.

E-mail address: dkim1@lsuhsc.edu

Oral Maxillofacial Surg Clin N Am 25 (2013) 61–66

http://dx.doi.org/10.1016/j.coms.2012.11.004

indwelling venous catheters. Despite the ingenuity of these novel technologies, clinical flap perfusion evaluation is still based on subjective criteria in both the intraoperative and postoperative periods. During surgery, evaluation of flow through a microvascular anastomosis has previously only been possible with the intraoperative clinical patency test (ie, strip test; **Fig. 1**), which has been reported to have a low sensitivity in the diagnosis of luminal obstruction.[2] Whether it is a pedicled flap or microvascular free-tissue transfer, early detection of vascular compromise with prompt correction still remains crucial to success of the procedure.

The ideal flap evaluation system for head and neck reconstructive surgeons would have a high sensitivity and high specificity for detecting compromised perfusion, and would have a high prognostic value for predicting vascular compromise and overall flap success. This ideal system would have the ability to distinguish between arterial and venous compromise and would also be able to predict future tissue necrosis. The introduction of intraoperative fluorescent angiography approaches the criteria listed earlier with a noninvasive, intraoperative system that is able to visualize blood flow and tissue perfusion.[3] With this system, assessment of anastomosis and vessel patency, along with soft tissue perfusion of the flap, is possible to help predict flap prognosis.

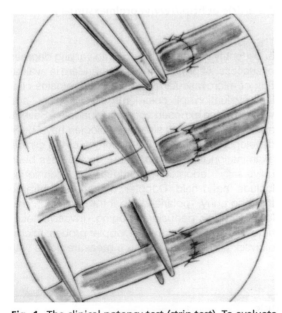

**Fig. 1.** The clinical patency test (strip test). To evaluate flow through a vessel, the vessel is occluded with 2 microvascular forceps downstream of the anastomosis. The distal forceps is gently moved more downstream while both forceps are still closed. The upstream forceps is then released and a patent anastomosis should allow blood to refill the area between the forceps.

## INDOCYANINE GREEN ANGIOGRAPHIC IMAGING SYSTEM

Intraoperative fluorescent angiographic imaging uses the dye indocyanine green (ICG) given intravenously through a peripheral vein. ICG is a water-soluble, tricarbocyanine dye and it has been used for more than 40 years for measuring cardiac output, as a liver function test, and for fluorescent angiography of the ocular choroidea.[4] ICG dye absorbs light in the near-infrared spectral range with a maximum at 805 nm and emits fluorescence with a maximum at 835 nm. These absorption and emission characteristics are optimal in the visualization of deeper structures because the absorption of intrinsic chromophores like hemoglobin and water is low in skin. This property makes skin transparent to ICG's emitted light spectrum and it can therefore be visualized and recorded with a suitable camera. This system uses near-infrared light projected onto the target area, where it penetrates deep into the skin and acts as an excitation light to the ICG dye and induces fluorescence from blood vessels containing dye within the deep dermal plexus and subcutaneous fat, rather than the superficial dermis as when fluorescein is used. Along with the emitted spectrum of light of ICG, this allows deeper vessel imaging than with fluorescein. Detection of blood vessels at a depth of up to 2 cm from the body surface has been shown.[5]

After intravascular injection of ICG, it is bound completely to large plasma proteins, allowing complete intravascular localization of the dye. The binding of the dye to these proteins makes it a suitable tracer for assessing vessel perfusion, because no capillary leakage of the dye occurs.[6] It also has a short half-life of 3 to 4 minutes, which allows sequential monitoring of skin perfusion because previous use does not affect subsequent examinations. ICG dye is efficiently removed from the blood by the liver and excreted into the bile. The incidence of adverse reactions after intravenous injection is low, and it has no effects on blood constituents or on the hemostatic system. Usual doses used for perfusion imaging are in the range of 0.1 to 1 mg/kg; toxicity is not reached when less than 5 mg/kg is used.

There are multiple near-infrared video camera systems that can be used for ICG angiography (ICGA). These systems include the SPY Elite system (LifeCell Corporation), the IC View System, and the PDE system (both from Pulsion Medical Systems and Hamamatsu Photonics). These imaging systems all activate ICG by emitting light at the appropriate wavelength (806 nm), which excites the dye to emit light at ~830 nm. The system uses a camera with appropriate filters to detect the fluorescent signals. ICG technology has also recently been integrated into the optical path of a surgical microscope that allows microangiography of vessels with diameters of less than 1 mm. It also allows for more magnified visualization of vascular flow through anastomosis sites.

## USE IN PEDICLED FLAPS

In pedicled flap surgery, adequate blood flow to the flap is an important determinant of the viability of soft tissue reconstruction. When flaps have localized or generalized hypoperfusion, they have a significant risk of postoperative wound dehiscence, skin slough or necrosis, infection, and flap loss. Until now, evaluation of flap perfusion has been based on subjective criteria that rely on tactile and visual characteristics including color, capillary refill, warmth, and bleeding. These subjective evaluations are often inaccurate even for the most experienced surgeons.

Other, more objective, evaluation tools have been proposed. These tools include ultrasonic Doppler, transcutaneous oxygen monitoring, and skin temperature recording, but none of these methods have been universally adopted because there is a lack of convincing evidence to their efficacy. ICGA is unique in that it is able to provide a dynamic map of dermal circulation that serves as a topographic analysis of the effective blood supply to the flap tissue.[7] It is also able to assess the surrounding normal tissue perfusion and compare that with the flap skin perfusion, providing a relative perfusion index (**Fig. 2**). Depending on the level of the perfusion differential, a low perfusion index may predict postoperative complications and partial or complete flap failure. At present, there are few data to establish a threshold for adequate perfusion. A perfusion index threshold value of 25% has been suggested, but it is not well established.[8,9] ICGA perfusion index measurements are merely a snapshot of the tissue perfusion at a given point in time; perfusion values for patients may fluctuate as a result of variations in systemic hemodynamics, cardiac output, body temperature, and administration of medications. Although no exact critical perfusion index value exists, a filling defect seen via ICGA on a pedicled flap during reconstruction may necessitate modification of the surgical plan to proactively prevent flap complications.

## USE IN MICROVASCULAR FREE-TISSUE TRANSFER

Microvascular free-tissue transfer has become a dependable reconstructive method for complex hard and soft tissue defects. Advances in surgical

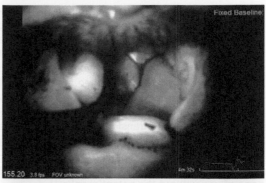
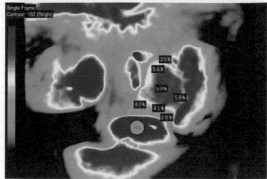

**Fig. 2.** (*Top*) Still image of video of inset soft tissue flap to the left mandible and buccal mucosa showing good, even distribution of fluorescence throughout the skin paddle of the flap. Close examination of the image reveals the deep dermal plexus. (*Bottom*) Use of proprietary software (SpyQ) allows evaluation of relative perfusion of the flap soft tissue compared with the unoperated area in the field of view (in this case, the lower lip).

instrumentation, suture materials, magnification, and technique have made this reconstructive method reliable. In the most experienced hands, there is currently a 1% to 5% risk of flap compromise that can lead to flap failure.[10] When microvascular free-tissue transfer reconstruction fails, it can produce an even larger tissue defect with surrounding necrosis. Even partial flap failure creates a difficult problem for the reconstructive surgeon. Thus, the search for an ideal technique to analyze flap perfusion and microsurgical anastomosis patency continues in an attempt to decrease the risk of postoperative flap compromise.

In microvascular free-tissue reconstruction, initial perfusion of the flap depends completely on the flow in the vascular pedicle. Techniques such as the double forceps patency tests and Doppler surveillance are used to assess the patency of the microvascular anastomosis. Subjective criteria such as color, capillary refill, and bleeding are used to assess the viability of transplanted tissue. Traditional radiographic contrast angiography is the standard for analysis of vascular anatomy. However, intraoperative angiography techniques using traditional intravenous contrast agents have proved cumbersome and add risks to the patient from the contrast dye. Radiation exposure to both the patient and the operating staff is also of concern. Traditional intraoperative angiography has therefore been considered largely inappropriate for free-tissue transfer. ICGA is a valuable tool for the microvascular reconstructive surgeon, because it provides the visual properties of traditional contrast angiography combined with relative ease of use without the potential risks.[11]

ICGA can provide important information at all stages of microvascular free-tissue transfer surgery. During harvest, it can provide information about the distribution of blood flow to the flap and the territories of tissue supplied by the vascular pedicle. This information is especially important when raising extended flaps for large, complex reconstructions. ICGA has also been shown in experimental and clinical studies to have a high sensitivity in identifying perforators and their supplied territory for use in perforator flaps.[12,13] The use of perforator flaps in microvascular free-tissue transfer has become favored because the perforator flap is based on 1 or 2 perforating vessels. Thus, sparing the inclusion of underlying fascia and muscle has permitted the reconstructive surgeon to decrease donor site morbidity, resulting in faster recovery for the patient. Disadvantages of the perforator flap are the high variability in perforator vessel anatomy and territories supplied. With the use of ICGA, the identification of the perforator and the territory it supplies can be verified before flap harvest, increasing the reliability and success rate of these types of flaps

(**Fig. 3**, Videos 1 and 2 [see videos online within this article at www.oralmaxsurgery.theclinics. com, February 2013 issue]).

ICGA also allows objective quality assessment of anastomotic patency, which is the primary determinant for initial microvascular free-flap survival (**Fig. 4**). Conventional subjective patency tests such as the double forceps test and clinical inspection have been shown to have a low sensitivity for revealing anastomotic deficiencies. As many as 22% of anastomoses classified as patent based on conventional subjective patency tests have shown abnormal flow through the anastomosis on subsequent angiographic studies.[14] Through the objective verification of the vascular inflow and outflow of the microvascular free-tissue flap, it would be possible to identify these vascular issues early, while the patient is still on the operating table. After the insetting and anastomosis of the vessels, the free-tissue flap can then be reanalyzed with ICGA to assess for adequacy of blood supply to all zones of the inset flap, which is especially important in preventing partial flap failure (Video 3 [see video online within this article at www.oralmaxsurgery.theclinics.com, February 2013 issue]).

ICGA has also found a role in patients undergoing reexploration surgery for a threatened blood supply to a microvascular free-tissue flap. Finding the cause of the flap compromise is essential in salvaging a microvascular free-tissue flap. These causes can be varied and include microvascular thrombosis, pedicle kinks, external compression of the vascular pedicle, hematoma, and vasospasm. In large reexploration studies, microvascular thrombosis is only found in half of the reexplored patients. Because early or very small

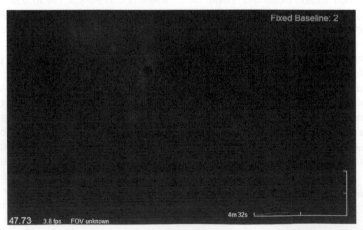

**Fig. 3.** Still image from Video 1. Right lower extremity intraoperative angiography before harvest of a fibula osteocutaneous flap. ICGA is used to identify the dominant perforator to the lateral calf skin to include it in the skin paddle of the flap.

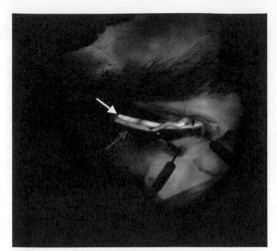

**Fig. 4.** Still image from Video 3. Intraoperative angiography of anterolateral thigh flap for a neurosurgical defect reconstruction anastomosed to the right superficial temporal vessels. Note complete filling of both artery (*red arrow*) and vein (*white arrow*).

microvascular thrombotic occlusions are hard to judge with subjective tests, a direct exploration of the anastomosis is almost always performed.[15,16] Given that only half of these threatened microvascular flaps have thrombotic occlusions, there is an overexploration of these microvascular anastomoses. Thus, the use of ICGA during reexploration surgery can significantly reduce the incidence of anastomosis revisions and prevent potentially harmful and unnecessary manipulation of the microvascular anastomosis when vascular flow is intact (Video 4 [see video online within this article at www.oralmaxsurgery.theclinics.com, February 2013 issue]).[10]

## SUMMARY

ICGA technology is increasingly being adopted by reconstructive surgeons for use in pedicle tissue flaps and microvascular free-tissue transfer procedures. This innovative technology provides an objective and quantifiable assessment of reconstruction that was not feasible only a few years ago. Many advantages for both the surgical team and the patient are obtained by the use of this technology. For the surgical team, peripheral intravenous access, ease of use, and the need for only minimal amounts of equipment make it advantageous. Patients are not exposed to unnecessary radiation, and minimal complications have been attributed to the administration of ICG dye. With the increasing adoption of this technology, the postoperative complication rate and the need for reoperation can be further decreased, making

these reconstructive procedures even more predictable. At present, the main disadvantage of this technology is its cost; with time and greater adoption of this technology, the cost will eventually decrease. Decreased postoperative complications and reduced need for revision surgery with the use of this technology will play a significant role in decreasing the overall health care costs for these complex reconstructive procedures.

## SUPPLEMENTARY DATA

Supplementary data related to this article can be found online at http://dx.doi.org/10.1016/j.coms. 2012.11.004.

## REFERENCES

1. Sloan G, Sasakie S. Non-invasive monitoring of tissue viability. Clin Plast Surg 1985;12:185–95.
2. Krag C, Holck S. The value of the patency test in microvascular anastomosis: correlation between observed patency and size of intraluminal thrombus: an experimental study in rats. Br J Plast Surg 1981; 34:64.
3. Holm C. Clinical applications of ICG fluorescence imaging in plastic and reconstructive surgery. Open Surg Oncol J 2010;2:37–47.
4. Flower RW, Hochheimer BF. Indocyanine green fluorescence and infrared absorption choroidal angiography performed simultaneously with fluorescein angiography. Johns Hopkins Med J 1976;138:33–42.
5. Still J, Law E, Dawson J, et al. Evaluation of the circulation of reconstructive flaps using laser-induced fluorescence of indocyanine green. Ann Plast Surg 1999;42:266–74.
6. Ishihara H, Otomo N, Suzuki A, et al. Detection of capillary protein leakage by glucose and indocyanine green dilutions during the early post-burn period. Burns 1998;24:525–31.
7. Holm C, Mayr M, Hofter E, et al. Perioperative assessment of skin viability using indocyanine green. Br J Plast Surg 2002;55:635–44.
8. Holzbach T, Taskov C, Henke J, et al. Evaluation of perfusion in skin flaps by laser induced indocyanine green fluorescence. Handchir Mikrochir Plast Chir 2005;37(6):396–402.
9. Giunta RE, Holzbach T, Taskov C, et al. Prediction of flap necrosis with laser induced indocyanine green fluorescence in a rat model. Br J Plast Surg 2005; 58(5):695–701.
10. Holm C, Dornseifer U, Sturtz G, et al. Sensitivity and specificity of ICG angiography in free flap reexploration. J Reconstr Microsurg 2010;26:311–6.
11. Pestana IA, Coan B, Erdmann D, et al. Early experience with fluorescent angiography in free-tissue

transfer reconstruction. Plast Reconstr Surg 2006; 117(1):37–43.

12. Mothes H, Donicke T, Friedel R, et al. Indocyanine-green fluorescence video angiography used clinically to evaluate tissue perfusion in microsurgery. J Trauma 2004;57(5):1018–24.

13. Mothes H, Dinkelaker T, Donicke T, et al. Outcome prediction in microsurgery by quantitative evaluation of perfusion using ICG fluorescence angiography. J Hand Surg Eur Vol 2009;34(2):238–46.

14. Holm C, Dornseifer U, Sturtz G, et al. The intrinsic transit time of free microvascular flaps: clinical and prognostic implications. Microsurgery 2010;30(2):91–6.

15. Chen KT, Mardini S, Chuang DC, et al. Timing of presentation of the first signs of vascular compromise dictates the salvage outcome of free flap transfers. Plast Reconstr Surg 2007;120:187–95.

16. Bui DT, Cordeiro PG, Hu QY, et al. Free flap exploration: indications, treatment, and outcomes in 1193 free flaps. Plast Reconstr Surg 2007;119:2092–100.

# Burning Mouth Syndrome

Heidi C. Crow, DMD, MS*, Yoly Gonzalez, DDS, MS, MPH

## KEYWORDS

• Burning mouth syndrome • Glossodynia • Stomatodynia

## KEY POINTS

• Burning mouth syndrome is a chronic disorder for which there are no standardized validated diagnostic criteria.
• Patients with burning mouth are often a challenge to manage, especially in a standard clinical surgery practice.
• Patients often do not report complete symptom resolution with single-modality therapy, frustrating even the best-intentioned clinician.
• A stepped treatment protocol initially using low-risk treatments followed by combination protocols appears to have the most support in the literature.

## INTRODUCTION

Many different terms have been used to describe a condition whereby the tongue or other intraoral areas develop "burning" type pain. If this affects the tongue it may be termed glossodynia, glosso-pyrosis or, less frequently, glossalgia. If it is more widespread, burning mouth syndrome (BMS), primary burning mouth, stomatodynia, and oropy-rosis have been used. Although there is some controversy as to whether glossopyrosis can be differentiated from oropyrosis,[1] current literature suggests that these oral complaints can be viewed as similar entities that may encompass only the tongue, lips, gingiva, palate, buccal mucosa, or a combination of these mucosal regions. Inherent in the diagnosis is an understanding that there are several systemic and local conditions that can lead to a sensation of burning pain in the mouth. If one of these conditions is responsible for causing the pain, after successful treatment of the underlying condition the burning pain will resolve.

This article focuses on descriptions, etiologic theories, and management of primary BMS, a condition for which underlying causative agents have been ruled out.

## DEFINITION

BMS is a chronic disorder for which there are no standardized validated diagnostic criteria. Various approaches to developing a consistent definition have been attempted by several organizations. The American Academy of Orofacial Pain[2] uses that of Sardella and colleagues,[3] in which the condition is described as a burning sensation in the oral mucosa occurring in the absence of clinically apparent mucosal abnormalities or laboratory findings, often perceived as painful; intrinsic to this definition is that the clinician has not observed any clinical abnormality in the oral cavity and that laboratory testing has ruled out systemic involvement.

The International Headache Society (ICHD-II)[4] describes Burning Mouth within Central Causes of Pain as an intraoral burning sensation for which no medical or dental cause can be found, and with the following diagnostic criteria: (1) pain in the mouth present daily and persisting for most of the day; (2) oral mucosa is of normal appearance; and (3) local and systemic diseases have been excluded, with an additional comment specifying that pain may be confined to the tongue (glossodynia). This condition has also been described by terms that

Department of Oral Diagnostic Sciences, University at Buffalo, 355 Squire Hall, 3435 Main Street, Buffalo, NY 14214, USA
* Corresponding author.
*E-mail address:* hccrow@buffalo.edu

Oral Maxillofacial Surg Clin N Am 25 (2013) 67–76
http://dx.doi.org/10.1016/j.coms.2012.11.001
1042-3699/13/$ – see front matter © 2013 Published by Elsevier Inc.

include stomatopyrosis, glossopyrosis, stomato-dynia, glossodynia, sore mouth, sore tongue, and oral dysesthesia.[5–7]

## CLINICAL CHARACTERISTICS

BMS is characterized by a burning sensation or other dysesthesia, with normal appearance of the oral mucosa. Multiple sites in the oral cavity may be affected, with the tongue being the most common; however, other areas of the intraoral mucosa may also be involved. BMS pain is usually bilateral and does not follow peripheral nerve distributions.

The pain associated with the condition has been described as continuous, with an intensity that is moderate to severe. Its daily pattern may fluctuate, often being better in the morning and more aggravating toward the evening; it rarely affects sleep. Associated symptoms may include alterations of taste (dysgeusia, hypogeusia) and smell, dry mouth (xerostomia) despite normal salivation, altered salivary composition,[8,9] and paresthesia. Mild food and noncarbonated beverages may improve the burning symptoms, but extremes of spice or temperature may worsen it.[10]

The diagnosis of primary BMS is purely clinical, and is based on patients' description of symptoms as well as on the exclusion of any systemic or local factors that may give rise to secondary burning sensations within the oral mucosa (and consequently a different diagnosis). These factors include endocrinopathies such as hypothyroidism,[11,12] diabetes,[13] oral candidiasis,[14] decreased salivation, secondary effects of drugs, and nutritional deficiencies.[15,16] Secondary BMS symptoms disappear with treatment of the underlying cause.

## EPIDEMIOLOGY

Several investigators have described BMS based on person, place, and time. The data from which clinical information has been obtained are limited to cross-sectional studies and convenience samples with heterogeneous composition, owing to the need for consensus on the diagnostic criteria. Population-based information is based on national surveys. Although symptom improvement has been reported over time,[17] there are no longitudinal data on the natural history or onset of the condition.

The prevalence of BMS symptoms in adults has been estimated at from 0.7% to 7.9%.[18,19] Symptoms worsen with an increase in age, have a female gender preference, and have been associated with menopause.[20–23] Some investigators have reported a prevalence as high as 40% on convenience samples.[24]

## CLASSIFICATION

A conventional and practical classification presented in the literature on burning mouth divides this condition into primary and secondary. As presented in **Table 1**, secondary BMS is associated with a preexisting condition or cause, and once such a condition is treated the symptoms improve or disappear.

## ETIOLOGY

The etiology and pathophysiology of primary BMS have remained largely unknown. Data from several experimental models support the hypothesis that primary BMS is a neuropathic condition.[23] The role of the peripheral and/or central nervous system(s) is supported by studies involving quantitative sensory testing and functional imaging methods.[23] **Table 2** illustrates the sensory neuropathic changes that have been associated with BMS.

Secondary burning mouth, unfortunately, has been associated with several local and systemic conditions (see **Table 1**). The clinical concern is that ruling out each of these possible related conditions to allow diagnosis of primary burning mouth is costly and time consuming. The role of the various causative factors is unknown, so it is difficult to develop a reasonable and solid scientifically supported protocol. In several studies, complete blood counts were done on all patients complaining of BMS; there is no indication, however, that abnormalities in complete blood count are associated with a burning sensation in the mouth. In patients with low but normal nutritional findings, there is no indication that additional supplementation of the nutritional substances will be absorbed, nor is there information regarding "how much is enough" for patients. A thorough clinical examination demonstrating normal appearance of mucosal tissues along with a careful review of systems may be indicated for clinically ruling out the various risk indicators associated with secondary burning mouth. Though not tested to date, it would be very illustrative to determine the rate of abnormal findings on laboratory testing in the presence of a normal examination and negative review of systems.

## PSYCHOLOGICAL FACTORS

It has been postulated that patients with BMS may have distinct psychological characteristics. Conditions such as depression, anxiety, and somatization[8,25] have been described in this population. In

**Table 1**
**Risk indicators for secondary BMS**

| Risk Indicators | Indications for Testing-History of: | Test for: |
|---|---|---|
| Fungal infection | Antibiotic use, tongue coating/erythema | Culture/swab |
| Nutritional deficiencies | Anemia, excessive bleeding, bulimia, vomiting, celiac disease, Crohn disease | Iron, vitamin B12, vitamin B-complex |
| Endocrine disorders | Polydipsia, polyphagia, polyuria, poor wound healing, infections, cold sensitivity, fatigue | Diabetes, hypothyroidism, hormone deficiency |
| Hyposalivation | Dry mouth | Sjögren syndrome, rheumatoid arthritis; review medications for xerostomic side effects |
| Medications | Medication use | Review medication list for angiotensin-converting enzyme inhibitor or antihyperglycemic side effects |
| Esophageal reflux | Heartburn, regurgitation | Refer to primary medical doctor |
| Taste disturbances | Dysgeusia, metallic taste | Taste acuity, detection of bitterness, reaction to acid/spicy tastes |
| Neuropathy or neuralgias | Sensory changes: hyperalgesia, hypo-/hyperesthesia | Refer to neurologist: brain imaging |
| Psychological factors | Depression, anxiety | Screen for depression, anxiety, somatization (Axis II evaluation). Refer to biobehavioral medicine |

addition, BMS patients are subjected to elevated psychological stress that is not necessarily associated with stressful life events. Intensity of burning sensation, however, is apparently not influenced by severity of psychological symptoms.[26,27] It has not been well documented whether the rate of occurrence of these psychological conditions is unique to BMS or consistent with other chronic pain conditions. In addition, these psychological conditions could be comorbidities, modifiers of the burning mouth condition, or a behavioral consequence of having BMS. Although the role

**Table 2**
**Theoretical models of causality for primary burning mouth syndrome (BMS)**

| Theoretical Model | Description |
|---|---|
| Dysfunction of the chorda tympani | Abnormal interplay between lingual and chorda tympani nerves |
| Small afferent fiber atrophy | Small fiber neurologic damage in the oral cavity |
| Upregulated TRPV1 receptor (Transient Receptor Potential Vanilloid type 1) | Increased number of heat and capsaicin receptors in nerve fibers, leading to release of sensory neuropeptides, promoting neurogenic inflammation |
| Central nervous system pain pathway and dopamine receptor | Altered central modulation. Decreased dopaminergic function. Decreased endogenous dopamine levels |
| Autoimmune disorders | BMS associated with lichen planus due to elevated expression of CD14 mRNA and decreased levels of TLR-2 mRNA in saliva |

*Data from* Suarez Dural P, Clark G. Burning mouth syndrome: an update on diagnosis and treatment methods. In: Clark GT, Dionne RA, editors. Orofacial pain: a guide to medications and management. New York: John Wiley & Sons; 2012. p. 232–46.

of psychiatric disorders in the pathophysiology of BMS is still unknown, these disorders must be actively elucidated because of their impact on quality of life.[28] Screening for psychiatric disorders may be relevant, because of its impact on treatment outcomes.[29] Appropriate management includes referral to health professionals who can assist these patients with their mental health status to provide a better quality of life.[30,31]

## MANAGEMENT OF BURNING MOUTH

Several systematic reviews that address the management of BMS have been published.[7,32,33] These reviews have highlighted the lack of randomized clinical trials that are available, as well as the limitations of many treatments when compared with placebo. **Table 3** lists randomized controlled trials of various oral and systemic therapies along with the side effects of treatment. With treatment regimens that range from topical, over-the-counter products to systemic medications with potentially significant side effects, the clinician is faced with treatment dilemmas that may not be easily answered even with the help of systematic reviews. This section considers a stepped treatment protocol, which highlights potential side effects and benefits of several published therapies.

When assessing treatment success, the calculation of number needed to treat (NNT) has been used to quantify relative success. The NNT, though originally designed to demonstrate reduction of adverse outcome based on providing an intervention,[34] has been used in determining the success of treatments for neuropathic pain.[35] In this calculation, the "success" of a treatment for pain needs to be defined, and previous reports have used more than 50% pain relief as a reasonable clinically relevant outcome.[35,36] This value, unfortunately, has not generally been reported in publications assessing treatments for BMS. Instead, statistically significant changes in pain in comparison with placebo have been used. Using a percent absolute risk reduction, calculated from subtracting the percent event rate with a drug from the percent event rate with the placebo, allowed Patton and colleagues[37] to calculate some values of NNT for treatments for BMS. Wherever available, the NNT for a treatment for burning mouth is reported in this section.

### Nonprescription Treatments

α-Lipoic acid has been used for diabetic neuropathy for many years, with support for its use in multiple studies including a meta-analysis comprising more than 1250 patients.[38] Because of its use with diabetic neuropathy, a protocol was developed and tested for BMS. A double-blind, randomized controlled trial using 200 mg of α-lipoic acid 3 times a day yielded significant improvement over placebo, with an NNT of 3.3.[39] Because of this and other supportive articles, Patton and colleagues classified α-lipoic acid as a "Class I" treatment whereby the benefit far outweighs the risk of use, with recommendation for administration of the treatment.[37] Subsequent to their review, additional studies have not yielded a statistical difference over placebo.[40–42] What should be appreciated in these studies, however, is the high rate of success of placebo and the large variations in pain response for both placebo and active trial groups. In general, all 3 of these studies yielded a decrease of 2 points on an 11-point visual analog scale (VAS), which in one of the studies yielded a 50% pain reduction in 30% of the patients.[40] In this study, however, Carbone and colleagues reported a greater than 50% pain reduction with 25% of patients on placebo, and similar or superior reductions in VAS occurred in the placebo groups in the other 2 studies. From a treatment standpoint, α-lipoic acid supplementation may help a limited number of patients, but not at a higher rate than placebo. As the risk is limited in otherwise healthy individuals and the cost of treatment is consistent with other nutritional supplements, a 2-month regimen could be considered in patients who otherwise would be considered for higher-cost or higher-risk treatment regimens.

Capsaicin, administered both topically and systemically, has been used for the treatment of BMS and other neuropathic conditions. Systemically administered capsaicin has showed success compared with placebo[43] in treating BMS, but carries a high risk of gastric pain (32% of subjects in the active treatment arm). Until recently, the lack of randomized controlled trials limited the ability to compare topical capsaicin results with those for placebo. Topical capsaicin had reported success in case trials,[44,45] and recent randomized controlled trials now indicate that it decreases pain rating when compared with placebo.[46,47] Adverse effects of capsaicin include an increase in burning sensation, which can lead to noncompliance. For treatment of post-herpetic neuralgia pain on dermal sites, pretreatment of the area with topical anesthetic was able to increase compliance in patients using a high-dose capsaicin patch.[48] In addition, animal research combining local anesthesia and capsaicin indicates that this may allow a more selective targeting of pain receptors in the trigeminal system.[49] Further research in these areas may provide

**Table 3**
**Randomized controlled trials of various oral or systemic therapies for burning mouth syndrome**

| Treatment | Warnings/Side Effects | Rate of Success | Reference |
|---|---|---|---|
| α-Lipoic acid | Hypoglycemic reactions; gastric upset | >50% pain reduction: 10/34 patients (no difference from placebo) | Carbone et al,[40] 2009 |
| | | Mean reduction of 2 points on 0–10 VAS (no difference from placebo) | López-Jornet et al,[31] 2008 |
| | | Mean reduction of 20 points on 0–100 VAS (no difference from placebo) | Cavalcanti et al,[42] 2009 |
| | | "decided improvement or resolution" 26/30 patients (significant difference from placebo) | Femiano et al,[39] 2002 |
| Capsaicin (topical) | Increased burning | Statistically significant mean reduction of 2 points on a 0–10 VAS with active treatment (no statistical difference seen with placebo) | Silvestre et al,[47] 2012 |
| | | Mean reduction of 3 points on 0–10 VAS (significant difference from placebo) | Marino et al,[46] 2010 |
| Capsaicin (systemic) | Gastric pain (32% in treatment arm) | VAS reported as significantly lower in the treated group compared with placebo. Unable to determine mean change | Petruzzi et al,[43] 2004 |
| Clonazepam (systemic 0.5 mg/d) | Dizziness, drowsiness, emotional liability | VAS reported as significantly lower than baseline in active group (mean reduction 3 points on a 0–10 VAS), but placebo group also had significant reduction (1.5 points on VAS). No statistical comparison between active and placebo treatment | Heckmann et al,[54] 2012 |
| Clonazepam (topical, 1 mg TID dissolve and expectorate) | | Significant difference from placebo with mean reduction of 2 points on 0–10 scale VAS over 2 wk with active treatment. Mean reduction in VAS with placebo 0.6 | Gremeau-Richard et al,[52] 2004 |
| Gabapentin (systemic) | Dizziness, drowsiness | Odds ratio for possibility of improvement or resolution: 7 times higher for α-lipoic acid 5.7 times higher for gabapentin 13.2 times higher for combination α-lipoic acid and gabapentin | López-D'Alessandro et al,[57] 2011 |

*Abbreviation:* VAS, visual analog scale.

evidence for the clinical practice of mixing capsa-icin with benzocaine for oral delivery in BMS and oral neuropathic pain. With relatively low cost and low risk in the topical formulation, capsaicin has demonstrated some success in 2 clinical trials, and should be considered for patients with BMS. Although no published studies have examined the use of capsaicin with topical anesthetic, this clinical practice could help with compliance and is starting to receive support for use with other types of neuropathic pain in other body sites.

Investigators have evaluated the use of St John's wort (Hypericum perforatum), but there is no evidence to support the use of this herbal compound as a treatment modality for BMS.[50]

## Prescription Treatments

Clonazepam, a benzodiazepine used for seizure control and panic disorder, has undergone off-label use for BMS for many years. It has been used systemically,[51] topically (dissolve and expec-torate),[52] and in combination.[53] Reported success rates in non–placebo-controlled regimens, using as the benchmark improvement of pain of greater than 50%, are as high as 80%.[53] In an earlier study, 70% of patients reported at least "some" reduction in pain; however, 27% of these patients elected to stop use of clonazepam for reasons that included its side effects.[51] A recent randomized controlled trial of systemic clonazepam demon-strated a significant reduction in pain with the active drug; however, there was also a significant reduction in pain with placebo.[54] Concerns with clonazepam include dizziness and drowsiness[55] (of particular concern in an elderly population), as well as potential withdrawal effects. Though a recognized treatment in management of BMS, the lack of randomized controlled trials with clona-zepam demonstrating a benefit beyond placebo and the risks associated with systemic use may warrant reserving this treatment for those who do not respond to other therapies.[55]

Gabapentin, also used for seizure control and post-herpetic neuralgia, is used extensively in neuropathic pain. An early case report indicated its potential for success in BMS,[56] but a subse-quent open-label trial did not demonstrate pain reduction over the course of the up to 6-week study.[57] A more recent randomized controlled trial that tested α-lipoic acid, gabapentin, and the combination of the two demonstrated an improve-ment in burning in 55% of those using α-lipoic acid alone, 50% improvement in those using gabapen-tin alone, and 70% improvement in those using a combination of α-lipoic acid and gabapentin.[58] Gabapentin as a single-use drug does not appear to have a high rate of success in BMS, but it may be helpful in combination with other treatments.

Tricyclic antidepressants (TCA) and serotonin-norepinephrine reuptake inhibitors (SNRI) have demonstrated pain relief in neuropathic pain.[59] Using diabetic neuropathic pain, amitriptyline yielded an NNT of 3 for at least 50% reduction of pain.[60] Placebo-controlled studies in BMS for these drugs, however, are lacking. In patients with BMS, a retrospective analysis demonstrated some success with TCAs in burning mouth,[61]

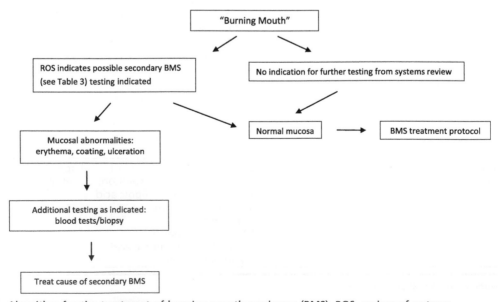

**Fig. 1.** Algorithm for the treatment of burning mouth syndrome (BMS). ROS, review of systems.

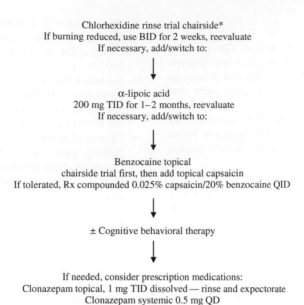

Chlorhexidine rinse trial chairside*
If burning reduced, use BID for 2 weeks, reevaluate
If necessary, add/switch to:

α-lipoic acid
200 mg TID for 1–2 months, reevaluate
If necessary, add/switch to:

Benzocaine topical
chairside trial first, then add topical capsaicin
If tolerated, Rx compounded 0.025% capsaicin/20% benzocaine QID

± Cognitive behavioral therapy

If needed, consider prescription medications:
Clonazepam topical, 1 mg TID dissolved — rinse and expectorate
Clonazepam systemic 0.5 mg QD
Gabapentin 300 mg QD (with concurrent α-lipoic acid 600 mg QD)
Tricyclic antidepressants

*Chlorhexidine rinse, with or without alcohol, has not been published as a treatment. Anecdotally, this
has provided relief for some patients and has allowed avoidance of higher-risk and higher-cost therapies.

**Fig. 2.** Treatment protocol for burning mouth syndrome. BID, twice a day; QD, once a day; QID, 4 times a day; Rx, treatment; TID, 3 times a day.

and a case report documented success with an SNRI.[62] Concerns with the use of these medications include dry mouth for amitriptyline (possibly compounding the oral complaints), significant cardiac rhythm issues, and sedation. The combination of potential side effects in an older population along with limited indications of their effectiveness limits the recommendation for use in BMS at this time.

### Biobehavioral Therapy

Cognitive behavioral therapy (which focuses on how beliefs and thoughts can influence behavior), used alone[63] or in combination with other therapies[64] for BMS, has shown success in reducing its intensity. Based on the evidence at the time, this therapy was recommended by Patton and colleagues[37] as a treatment that should be performed. A randomized controlled trial of group psychotherapy versus a placebo tablet resulted in a higher percentage of improvement in the patients receiving group therapy (70.8% improved) as opposed to those receiving placebo medication (40% improved).[65] With indications that biobehavioral therapy may increase the success achieved by other treatments or demonstrate improvement as a stand-alone therapy, it should be considered for use, especially in individuals whose medical conditions increase the risks associated with alternative therapies.

### SUMMARY

Many of the current etiologic theories of primary BMS focus on neuropathology. Unfortunately, not all treatment modalities that seem helpful in other neuropathic conditions appear to be successful in BMS. These patients are often a challenge to manage, especially in a standard clinical surgery practice. Patients often do not report complete symptom resolution with single-modality therapy, frustrating even the best-intentioned clinician.

Given the controversial nature of the disorder, a stepped treatment protocol initially using low-risk treatments followed by combination protocols appears to have the most support in the literature. Because of the relatively low prevalence of primary BMS, research should focus on developing multicenter trials that follow standard diagnostic protocols and use randomized controlled trials, to develop treatment protocols for clinical use. In the interim, the clinician may provide some relief from this difficult-to-manage condition using the best available information (**Figs. 1** and **2**).

## REFERENCES

1. Henkin RI, Gouliouk V, Fordyce A. Distinguishing patients with glossopyrosis from those with oropyrosis based upon clinical differences and differences in saliva and erythrocyte magnesium. Arch Oral Biol 2012;57(2):205–10.

2. de Leeuw R, editor. Orofacial Pain: Guidelines for Assessment, Diagnosis, and Management. Fourth Edition. Hanover Park, IL: Quintessence Publishing Co; 2008.

3. Sardella A, Lodi G, Demarosi F, et al. Causative or precipitating aspects of burning mouth syndrome: a case-control study. J Oral Pathol Med 2006; 35(8):466–71.

4. Headache Classification Subcommittee of the International Headache Society. The international classification of headache disorders: 2nd edition. Cephalalgia 2004;24(Suppl 1):9–160.

5. Merskey H, Bogduk N, editors. Classification of chronic pain. Second Edition. IASP Task Force on Taxonomy, Seattle: IASP Press; 1994.

6. Brufau-Redondo C, Martín-Brufau R, Corbalán-Velez R, et al. Burning mouth syndrome. Actas Dermo-Sifiliográficas (English Edition) 2008;99(6): 431–40 [in Spanish].

7. Zakrzewska JM, Forssell H, Glenny AM. Interventions for the treatment of burning mouth syndrome: a systematic review. J Orofac Pain 2003;17(4):293–300.

8. Granot M, Nagler RM. Association between regional idiopathic neuropathy and salivary involvement as the possible mechanism for oral sensory complaints. J Pain 2005;6(9):581–7.

9. Minor JS, Epstein JB. Burning mouth syndrome and secondary oral burning. Otolaryngol Clin North Am 2011;44(1):205–19.

10. Torgerson RR. Burning mouth syndrome. Dermatol Ther 2010;23(3):291–8.

11. Femiano F, Lanza A, Buonaiuto C, et al. Burning mouth syndrome and burning mouth in hypothyroidism: proposal for a diagnostic and therapeutic protocol. Oral Surg Oral Med Oral Pathol Oral Radiol Endod 2008;105(1):e22–7.

12. Femiano F, Gombos F, Esposito V, et al. Burning mouth syndrome (BMS): evaluation of thyroid and taste. Med Oral Patol Oral Cir Bucal 2006;11(1):E22–5.

13. Moore PA, Guggenheimer J, Orchard T. Burning mouth syndrome and peripheral neuropathy in patients with type 1 diabetes mellitus. J Diabetes Complications 2007;21(6):397–402.

14. Terai H, Shimahara M. Glossodynia from Candida-associated lesions, burning mouth syndrome, or mixed causes. Pain Med 2010;11(6):856–60.

15. Cho GS, Han MW, Lee B, et al. Zinc deficiency may be a cause of burning mouth syndrome as zinc replacement therapy has therapeutic effects. J Oral Pathol Med 2010;39(9):722–7.

16. De Giuseppe R, Novembrino C, Guzzi G, et al. Burning mouth syndrome and vitamin B12 deficiency. J Eur Acad Dermatol Venereol 2011;25(7): 869–70.

17. Sardella A, Lodi G, Demarosi F, et al. Burning mouth syndrome: a retrospective study investigating spontaneous remission and response to treatments. Oral Dis 2006;12(2):152–5.

18. Tammiala-Salonen T, Hiidenkari T, Parvinen T. Burning mouth in a Finnish adult population. Community Dent Oral Epidemiol 1993;21(2):67–71.

19. Ship JA, Grushka M, Lipton JA, et al. Burning mouth syndrome: an update. J Am Dent Assoc 1995; 126(7):842–53.

20. Bergdahl M, Bergdahl J. Burning mouth syndrome: prevalence and associated factors. J Oral Pathol Med 2007;28(8):350–4.

21. Ben Aryeh H, Gottlieb I, Ish-Shalom S, et al. Oral complaints related to menopause. Maturitas 1996; 24(3):185–9.

22. Maresky LS, van der Bijl P, Gird I. Burning mouth syndrome. Evaluation of multiple variables among 85 patients. Oral Surg Oral Med Oral Pathol 1993; 75(3):303–7.

23. Jääskeläinen SK. Pathophysiology of primary burning mouth syndrome. Clin Neurophysiol 2012; 123(1):71–7.

24. Rouleau T, Shychuk A, Kayastha J, et al. A retrospective, cohort study of the prevalence and risk factors of oral burning in patients with dry mouth. Oral Surg Oral Med Oral Pathol Oral Radiol Endod 2011;111:720–5.

25. Hakeberg M. Burning mouth syndrome: experiences from the perspective of female patients. Eur J Oral Sci 2003;111:305–11.

26. Firas AM, Quran AL. Psychological profile in burning mouth syndrome. Oral Surg Oral Med Oral Pathol Oral Radiol Endod 2004;97(3):339–44.

27. Bogetto F, Maina G, Ferro G, et al. Psychiatric comorbidity in patients with burning mouth syndrome. Psychosom Med 1998;60(3):378–85.

28. deSouza FT, Santos TP, Bernardes VF, et al. The impact of burning mouth syndrome on health-related quality of life. Health Qual Life Outcomes 2011;9(1):57.

29. Lamey P, Murray B, Eddle S, et al. The secretion of parotid saliva as stimulated by 10% citric acid is not related to precipitating factors in burning mouth syndrome. J Oral Pathol Med 2001;30: 121–4.

30. deSouza FT, Teixeira AL, Amaral TM, et al. Psychiatric disorders in burning mouth syndrome. J Psychosom Res 2012;72(2):142–6.

31. López-Jornet P, Camacho-Alonso F, Lucero-Berdugo M. Quality of life in patients with burning mouth syndrome. J Oral Pathol Med 2008;37(7): 389–94.

32. Martin WJ, Forouzanfar T. The efficacy of anticonvulsants on orofacial pain: a systematic review. Oral Surg Oral Med Oral Pathol Oral Radiol Endod 2011;111(5):627–33.

33. List T, Axelsson S, Leijon G. Pharmacologic interventions in the treatment of temporomandibular disorders, atypical facial pain, and burning mouth syndrome. A qualitative systematic review. J Orofac Pain 2003;17(4):301–10.

34. Cook RJ, Sackett DL. The number needed to treat: a clinically useful measure of treatment effect. BMJ 1995;310(6977):452–4.

35. Finnerup NB, Otto M, McQuay HJ, et al. Algorithm for neuropathic pain treatment: An evidence based proposal. Pain 2005;118(3):289–305.

36. McQuay HJ, Tramèr M, Nye BA, et al. A systematic review of antidepressants in neuropathic pain. Pain 1996;68(2–3):217–27.

37. Patton LL, Siegel MA, Benoliel R, et al. Management of burning mouth syndrome: systematic review and management recommendations. Oral Surg Oral Med Oral Pathol Oral Radiol Endod 2007;103:S39.e1–39.e13.

38. Ziegler D, Nowak H, Kempler P, et al. Treatment of symptomatic diabetic polyneuropathy with the antioxidant alpha-lipoic acid: a meta-analysis. Diabetic Medicine 2004;21(2):114–21.

39. Femiano F, Scully C. Burning mouth syndrome (BMS): double blind controlled study of alpha-lipoic acid (thioctic acid) therapy. J Oral Pathol Med 2002;31(5):267–9.

40. Carbone M, Pentenero M, Carrozzo M, et al. Lack of efficacy of alpha-lipoic acid in burning mouth syndrome: a double-blind, randomized, placebo-controlled study. Eur J Pain 2009;13(5):492–6.

41. Lopez-Jornet P, Camacho-Alonso F, Leon-Espinosa S. Efficacy of alpha lipoic acid in burning mouth syndrome: a randomized, placebo-treatment study. J Oral Rehabil 2009;36(1):52–7.

42. Cavalcanti DR, Da Silveira FR. Alpha lipoic acid in burning mouth syndrome—a randomized double-blind placebo-controlled trial. J Oral Pathol Med 2009;38(3):254–61.

43. Petruzzi M, Lauritano D, De Benedittis M, et al. Systemic capsaicin for burning mouth syndrome: short-term results of a pilot study. J Oral Pathol Med 2004;33(2):111–4.

44. Epstein JB, Marcoe JH. Topical application of capsaicin for treatment of oral neuropathic pain and trigeminal neuralgia. Oral Surg Oral Med Oral Pathol 1994;77(2):135–40.

45. Spice R, Hagen NA. Capsaicin in burning mouth syndrome: titration strategies. J Otolaryngol 2004;33(1):53–4.

46. Marino R, Torretta S, Capaccio P, et al. Different therapeutic strategies for burning mouth syndrome: preliminary data. J Oral Pathol Med 2010;39(8):611–6.

47. Silvestre F, Silvestre-Rangil J, Tamarit-Santafe C, et al. Application of a capsaicin rinse in the treatment of burning mouth syndrome. Med Oral Patol Oral Cir Bucal 2012;17:e1–4.

48. Webster LR, Peppin JF, Murphy FT, et al. Tolerability of NGX-4010, a capsaicin 8% patch, in conjunction with three topical anesthetic formulations for the treatment of neuropathic pain. J Pain Res 2012;5:7–13.

49. Kim HY, Kim K, Li HY, et al. Selectively targeting pain in the trigeminal system. Pain 2010;150(1):29–40.

50. Sardella A, Lodi G, Demarosi F, et al. *Hypericum perforatum* extract in burning mouth syndrome: a randomized placebo-controlled study. J Oral Pathol Med 2008;37(7):395–401.

51. Grushka M, Epstein J, Mott A. An open-label, dose escalation pilot study of the effect of clonazepam in burning mouth syndrome. Oral Surg Oral Med Oral Pathol Oral Radiol Endod 1998;86:557–61.

52. Gremeau-Richard C, Woda A, Navez M, et al. Topical clonazepam in stomatodynia: a randomised placebo-controlled study. Pain 2004;108(1–2):51–7.

53. Amos K, Yeoh SC, Farah CS. Combined topical and systemic clonazepam therapy for the management of burning mouth syndrome: a retrospective pilot study. J Orofac Pain 2011;25(2):125–30.

54. Heckmann SM, Kirchner E, Grushka M, et al. A Double-Blind Study on Clonazepam in Patients With Burning Mouth Syndrome. Laryngoscope 2012;122:813–6.

55. Ko JY, Kim MJ, Lee SG, et al. Outcome predictors affecting the efficacy of clonazepam therapy for the management of burning mouth syndrome (BMS). Arch Gerontol Geriatr 2012;55(3):755–61.

56. White TL, Kent PF, Kurtz DB, et al. Effectiveness of gabapentin for treatment of burning mouth syndrome. Arch Otolaryngol Head Neck Surg 2004;130(6):786–8.

57. Heckmann S, Heckmann J, Ungethüm A, et al. Gabapentin has little or no effect in the treatment of burning mouth syndrome—results of an open-label pilot study. Eur J Neurol 2006;13(7):e6–7.

58. López-D'alessandro E, Escovich L. Combination of alpha lipoic acid and gabapentin, its efficacy in the treatment of burning mouth syndrome: a randomized, double-blind, placebo controlled trial. Med Oral Patol Oral Cir Bucal 2011;16(5):e635–40.

59. Dworkin RH, O'Connor AB, Audette J, et al. Recommendations for the pharmacological management of neuropathic pain: an overview and literature update. Mayo Clin Proc 2010;85(Suppl 3):S3–14.

60. Smith HS, Argoff CE. Pharmacological treatment of diabetic neuropathic pain. Drugs 2011;71(5):557–89.

61. Pinto A, Sollecito T, DeRossi S. Burning mouth syndrome. A retrospective analysis of clinical characteristics and treatment outcomes. N Y State Dent J 2003;69(3):18–24.

62. Mignogna MD, Adamo D, Schiavone V, et al. Burning mouth syndrome responsive to duloxetine: a case report. Pain Med 2011;12(3):466–9.

63. Bergdahl J, Anneroth G, Perris H. Cognitive therapy in the treatment of patients with resistant burning mouth syndrome: a controlled study. J Oral Pathol Med 1995;24(5):213–5.

64. Femiano F, Gombos F, Scully C. Burning mouth syndrome: open trial of psychotherapy alone, medication with alpha-lipoic acid (thioctic acid), and combination therapy. Med Oral 2004;9(1):8–13.

65. Miziara ID, Filho BC, Oliveira R, et al. Group psychotherapy: an additional approach to burning mouth syndrome. J Psychosom Res 2009;67(5):443–8.

# Current Management Strategies for Verrucous Hyperkeratosis and Verrucous Carcinoma

James J. Sciubba, DMD, PhD[a,b,c,d], Joseph I. Helman, DMD[e,*]

## KEYWORDS

- Verrucous carcinoma • Proliferative verrucous leukoplakia • Hyperkeratosis

## KEY POINTS

- Verrucous carcinoma is a progressive lesion with high recurrence and high 5-year survival rates.
- It has a low incidence of bone invasion and cervical node metastasis is unusual.
- Most proliferative verrucous leukoplakia cases begin as homogeneous smooth plaques of leukoplakia that slowly increase in surface area to involve other areas either in continuity or anatomically separated, ultimately assuming a multifocal distribution.
- Surgery remains the preferred treatment.
- Further investigation into the combination of surgery and antiviral agents may bring additional improvement in patient care.

## INTRODUCTION

Since Hansen and colleagues[1] defined the term *proliferative verrucous leukoplakia* (PVL) in 1985, many reviews and reports of this unusual form of oral leukoplakia have been published. Before this study, the term *oral florid papillomatosis* was used to describe and characterize PVL.[2] More recently, the term *proliferative multifocal leukoplakia* was suggested to emphasize the early proliferative and multifocal nature of this entity and to indicate that initial manifestations are not warty or verrucous. When they finally become so, they histologically correspond to verrucous carcinoma, much as in the earlier descriptions by Batsakis and colleagues.[3,4] They emphasized that so-called verrucous hyperplasia was a precursor to verrucous carcinoma, conventional squamous cell carcinoma, and possibly papillary squamous carcinoma.

In a similar fashion, Shear and Pindborg[5] coined the term *verrucous hyperplasia* in 1980, which would represent PVL according to the currently accepted criteria for its definition. In their series of cases, they reported a 39% incidence of either squamous cell carcinoma or verrucous carcinoma, and microscopic evidence of dysplasia in 66% of cases.

Silverman and colleagues[6] subsequently published a large series of cases in which a subset of patients presenting with verrucous hyperplasia demonstrated a similar high rate of malignant transformation. Furthermore, a 100% transformation

[a] Department of Otolaryngology-Head and Neck Surgery, The Johns Hopkins Hospital, 600 North Wolfe Street, Sheikh Zayed Tower, Baltimore, MD 21287, USA; [b] Department of Pathology, The Johns Hopkins Hospital, 600 North Wolfe Street, Sheikh Zayed Tower, Baltimore, MD 21287, USA; [c] Department of Dermatology, The Johns Hopkins Hospital, 600 North Wolfe Street, Sheikh Zayed Tower, Baltimore, MD 21287, USA; [d] The Milton J. Dance Jr, Head and Neck Cancer Center, Greater Baltimore Medical Center, 6569 North Charles Street, Baltimore, MD 21204, USA; [e] Department of Oral and Maxillofacial Surgery, Taubman Center, University of Michigan, 1500 East Medical Center Drive, Room B1-B208, Ann Arbor, MI 48109-5018, USA
* Corresponding author.
*E-mail address:* jihelman@umich.edu

Oral Maxillofacial Surg Clin N Am 25 (2013) 77–82
http://dx.doi.org/10.1016/j.coms.2012.11.008
1042-3699/13/$ – see front matter © 2013 Elsevier Inc. All rights reserved.

rate was reported by Zakrzewska and colleagues[7] and Cabay and colleagues.[8]

The cause of this clinical entity remains obscure. There is an anatomic and gender predilection, poor response to treatment, and a significant risk for progression to verrucous carcinoma or invasive squamous cell carcinoma. This condition comprises a histologic continuum from hyperkeratosis to carcinoma, and neither attempts at prevention nor clinical intervention yield predictable results. Of importance is the notion that PVL remains a clinically based diagnosis without specific histologic connotation in the same fashion as typical oral leukoplakia.

From a demographic perspective, PVL is significantly more common in elderly women from age 62 to older than 70 years, as noted reported by Bagan and colleagues[9] and Silverman and colleagues,[6] with those cases reporting a long history of lesions characterized as leukoplakia.

## ETIOLOGY

PVL has no known origin. Unlike typical oral leukoplakia, PVL is more commonly noted in individuals without the usual risk factors of smoking, other forms of tobacco use, and excess alcohol consumption. Fungal and viral origins have not been proven, although earlier studies suggested that human papilloma virus (HPV) was of significance.[10,11] More recently, however, the relationship between PVL and oncogenic HPV has been challenged.[12–14] In contrast, Beltiol and colleagues[15] identified HPV in 100% of the patients with PVL, but in only 8.75% of the group without mucosal lesions. Clearly, the role of HPV in the origin of oral PVL remains undetermined.

Any site in the oral cavity may be involved with these lesions, but the most commonly affected areas, in descending orders of frequency, are the alveolar ridge, tongue, buccal mucosa, attached gingiva, floor of mouth, gingival sulcus, labial mucosa, and hard and soft palate.

From a genetic standpoint, PVL has been shown to demonstrate cell cycle alterations secondary to dysregulation of p16INK4a and p14ARF genes. Homozygous deletions, loss of heterozygosity, and mutational changes have been frequently shown. Although ploidy alterations have been considered a tool to predict malignant transformation, some have questioned this on the grounds of data validity.[16,17] High expression of cell cycle proteins Mcm-2 and Mcm-5 could help predict the long-term behavior and risk of malignant transformation of PVL. These markers could be useful diagnostic tools, superior to the Ki-67 proliferation marker.[18]

## CLINICAL PRESENTATION

Most PVL cases begin as homogeneous smooth plaques of leukoplakia that slowly increase in surface area to involve other areas either in continuity or anatomically separated, ultimately assuming a multifocal distribution (**Figs. 1–3**). The authors' combined anecdotal experience confirms the essential unifocal initial presentation, apparent inexorable progress to the more typical multifocal distribution, and the associated high rate of dysplasia or invasive cancer developing over a few years. In a reported large series, the alveolar ridge is most frequently affected, followed by the tongue and buccal mucosa (**Table 1**).

## DIAGNOSIS AND HISTOPATHOLOGY

A working diagnosis of proliferative leukoplakia is clinically based. It is supported by the progression

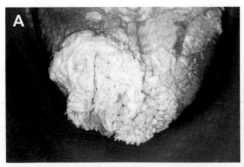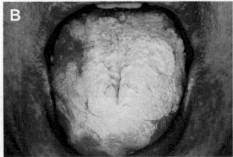

**Fig. 1.** (*A*) Broadly distributed lesions of proliferative verrucous leukoplakia over the dorsum of the tongue with variable surface textural features, including homogeneous, fissured, and prominent verrucous features. Microscopically, the features were reported as "consistent with verrucous carcinoma." (*B*) Persistent leukoplakia after conservative surgical resection approximately 14 months earlier. Moderately developed verrucous qualities are evident on either side of the midline, whereas toward the periphery a thinner more homogeneous pattern of keratinization is seen.

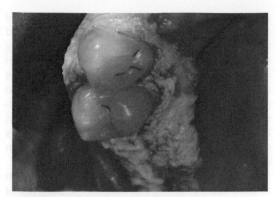

**Fig. 2.** Alveolar ridge PVL had developed over several months in this 68-year-old woman with no associated risk factors for oral cancer development. Verrucous carcinoma was diagnosed.

**Table 1**
**Site predilection and frequency**

| Location | Frequency |
| --- | --- |
| Alveolar ridge | 66.6% |
| Tongue | 50% |
| Buccal mucosa | 41.6% |
| Gingiva | 33.3% |
| Oral floor | 25% |
| Gingival sulcus | 25% |
| Labial mucosa | 16.6% |
| Hard & soft palate | 8.3% each |

*Data from* Gouvea AF, Vargas PA, Coletta RD, et al. Clinicopathologic features and immune histochemical expression of p53, Ki-67, Mcm-2 and Mcm-5 in proliferative verrucous leukoplakia. J Oral Pathol 2010;39:447–52.

from initially smooth, uniform, and homogeneous lesions to those that are granular, and finally to warty or verrucous lesions with an erythematous or erythroplastic component. The latter features develop over a variable time frame without intervention, and often in a multifocal distribution.

The pathologic nature of this entity is characterized by variation from one area to another within the region being sampled when an incisional biopsy is performed. It has been noted by way of general experience, and reported in the literature, that a wide range of abnormality can be found, from simple benign hyperkeratosis to invasive squamous cell carcinoma. Other forms of abnormality include ranges of dysplasia, verrucous hyperplasia, verrucous carcinoma, and, uncommonly, papillary squamous cell carcinoma.[1,4,19]

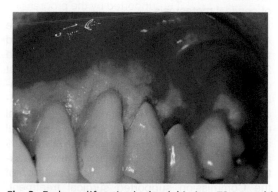

**Fig. 3.** Early proliferative leukoplakia in a 72-year-old man without exposure to tobacco or significant alcohol use. The maxillary arch was uniformly involved by this process, which began as a smooth surface alteration 2 years earlier. Histologically this was characterized as a benign minimally papillary hyperkeratosis.

## TREATMENT
### Photodynamic Therapy

The concept of photodynamic therapy is based on the activation of a photosensitizer by light of various wavelengths on superficial malignant or premalignant lesions. The photosensitizer is administered systemically, generating cytotoxic effects when the cells are exposed to light. One of the significant limitations of PDT is the marginal depth of penetration to the cutaneous or mucosal level.

Hematoporphyrin (Photofrin) was used initially at the Mayo Clinic in 1960 by Lipson and Schwartz.[20] They observed that administration of hematoporphyrin generated fluorescence of neoplastic lesions; this was used during surgery for tumor detection.[20]

One of the targets of photodamage by Photofrin was the mitochondria of cells, with no accumulation in the nuclei. This process resulted in diminished risk for DNA mutation or additional carcinogenesis. In addition to targeting the tumor cells, however, PDT has an effect on the microvasculature of the tumor bed and the inflammatory and immune systems, resulting in apoptosis and tumor control.[21] Photodynamic therapy has been effective in ablation of early superficial lesions of head and neck cancers, with up to 75% of the complete responses sustained at 2 years.[22]

Although PDT has been a viable treatment option, the side effects of dihematoporphyrin ether include hypersensitive skin reactions, local edema, nausea, and liver toxicity. Skin photosensitivity may last for up to 14 weeks; therefore, a topical option with fewer side effects was investigated. Topical application of 5-aminolevulinic acid activated with a 585-nm pulsed dye laser showed a 78% average reduction of laryngeal keratosis, with no significant differences between the outpatient and the operating room settings. Aminolevulinic acid (ALA) is not a photosensitizer but rather a precursor of protoporphyrin in the heme biosynthesis pathway.[23]

Chen and colleagues[24] evaluated ALA in the management of 8 oral verrucous hyperplasia and 24 oral leukoplakia lesions. All 8 oral verrucous hyperplastic lesions were treated weekly and showed complete response after an average of 3.8 treatments. No recurrence was seen within a mean follow-up of 10.6 months. The oral leukoplakia lesions were treated twice a week (because of limited response in a previous study administering topical ALA and PDT once a week). Complete response was achieved in 8 and partial response in 16 lesions after an average of 3.5 treatments. Of the 8 complete responses in the oral leukoplakia group, 2 recurred after 9 and 11 months. The remaining 6 complete responses showed no evidence of relapse after a mean follow-up period of 7.2 months.

Chen and colleagues[25] also reported the case of a patient with verrucous carcinoma in the commissure of the lip; the patient was a smoker and areca quid chewer also treated with ALA and PDT. The lesion showed complete remission in the extraoral aspect of the lip after 6 treatments and after 22 treatments to the intraoral tumor. No recurrence was identified after 6 months of follow-up.

Enough evidence exists to initiate treatment of PVL, and possibly even verrucous carcinoma, using photodynamic therapy. Longer follow-up and further identification of dosage and regimens, along with well-designed prospective randomized clinical trials are necessary to give additional validity to this treatment modality.

## Surgery

Surgery has been considered the preferred treatment for PVL and verrucous carcinoma, but the recurrence rate for both types of lesions has been high. This finding calls into question the operative management of the disease.

Walvekar and colleagues[26] reported on 101 oral verrucous carcinomas treated with surgery; 68% of the patients experienced local recurrence. On univariate analysis, tumor location (in the upper alveolar-palatal complex), presence of a premalignant lesion (ie, leukoplakia or submucous fibrosis), smoking, and positive margins were statistically significant for worse outcomes. The overall disease-free survival with surgical therapy was 77.6%. The incidences of cervical node metastasis and tumor invading bone were extremely low, consistent with data from Oliveira and colleagues.[27]

Femiano and colleagues[28] reported similar recurrence rates after excision of PVL. This study prospectively and randomly assigned 2 groups of 25 patients with HPV+ PVL paired and matched to 2 different treatment modalities. Group A was treated with surgical scalpel excision with normal surrounding mucosa, whereas Group B was treated with similar surgery in addition to Viruxan (methisoprinol), a synthetic agent with immuno-modulatory properties and antiviral activity against HPV. After 18 months of follow-up, 18 recurrences (72%) were seen in Group A compared with 4 relapses (16%) in Group B.

Surgical resection may be the intuitive approach to eliminate the lesion, but the biologic behavior of PVL and verrucous carcinoma probably requires addressing the possible underlying viral infection, if it exists, in addition to the excisional procedure.

## Radiation Therapy

For a long time there was a perception that radiotherapy changed the biologic behavior of verrucous carcinoma into a more aggressive squamous cell carcinoma.

In 1988, Nair and colleagues[29] reported on 52 cases of oral verrucous carcinoma treated with radiation. Fifteen patients with well-circumscribed T1 through T2 and early T3 lesions were treated with interstitial brachytherapy with single plane radium implants. Thirteen (87%) of the 15 patients treated with brachytherapy were alive with no evidence of disease after 3 years. Eight (25%) of 31 patients treated with external radiation survived, disease-free. The difference in survival rates may have been related to selection bias. The group receiving brachytherapy had smaller tumors with negative cervical node metastasis, whereas the group receiving external-beam radiation had larger tumors and a high incidence of cervical metastasis.

A report by the Commission on Cancer at the American College of Surgeons in 2001 reviewed the National Cancer database and identified 2350 cases of verrucous carcinoma. The most common treatment was surgery alone (69.7%), followed by surgery with irradiation (11%), and irradiation alone (10.3%). The 5-year relative survival rate was 77.9%. For localized disease, survival after surgery was 88.9% compared with 57.6% after irradiation. The rate of anaplastic transformation after irradiation was 6.7%. The conclusion of the Commission supported surgical treatment, especially for cases originating in the oral cavity.[30]

## Laser Ablation

The authors did not find evidence of reliable data on laser ablation when compared with surgical excision or just the "wait and see" approach in the management of PVL.

Although oral leukoplakia likely has a different origin and progression, one group compared laser ablation versus the wait-and-see approach in 200 patients (100 patients in each group) and followed them for 10 years. They didn't find differences in outcomes between the treatment group and the control group.[31]

In the case of verrucous lesions, the authors believe that laser ablation eliminates the ability to identify whether the lesion had any area of invasive squamous cell carcinoma, and therefore they do not advocate its use.

### Medical Management: Chemoprevention

Initial data from MD Anderson Cancer Center in the early 1980s supported the use of cancer chemoprevention through administering systemic 13-*cis*-retinoic acid to patients with premalignant lesions.[32]

Only recently a study reported the result in 2 small groups of patients with PVL treated with either topical or systemic retinoid therapy. The evaluators of the outcomes were blinded to the treatment modality. Eleven patients were treated with systemic retinoids and 5 with topical; 1 received both topical and systemic therapy. Seven lesions (6 in the systemic treatment group and 1 in the topical) improved, but 7 became worse (5 in the systemic therapy group and 2 in the topical group); the balance remained unchanged.[33] Although the study was preliminary, the results suggest a possible role for prospective chemoprevention studies in PVL. These studies should address the proposed viral association with PVL and verrucous carcinoma, especially considering that the combination of surgery and antiviral agents showed significant success.[28]

### SUMMARY

Proliferative verrucous leukoplakia, a lesion of unknown origin and with no strictly defined diagnostic criteria, is worthy of great clinical concern and scrutiny. The rate of malignant transformation associated with this entity was as high as 74% in one series.[11]

A wide range of pathologic findings characterize the clinically diverse presentation and slow evolution of the stated abnormalities. Treatment options are varied, with no consensus regarding the most efficient and effective strategy. Further complicating the unusual biology and behavior of this lesion is the usual multifocal presentation and progression observed, with lifelong vigilance required after treatment.

Verrucous carcinoma is a progressive lesion with high recurrence and 5-year survival rates. It has a low incidence of bone invasion, and cervical node metastasis is unusual. Surgery is still the preferred treatment. Further investigation into the combination of surgery and antiviral agents may bring additional improvement in patient care.

### REFERENCES

1. Hansen LS, Olson JA, Silverman S Jr. Proliferative verrucous leukoplakia. A long-term study of thirty patients. Oral Surg Oral Med Oral Pathol 1985; 60(3):285–98.
2. van der Waal I, Reichart PA. Oral proliferative verrucous hyperplasia revisited. Oral Oncol 2008;44:719–21.
3. Aguirre JM. Proliferative multifocal leukoplakia better name than proliferative verrucous leukoplakia. World J Surg Oncol 2011;9:122–3.
4. Batsakis JG, Suarez P, el-Naggar AL. Proliferative leukoplakia and its related lesions. Oral Oncol 1999;35(4):354–9.
5. Shear M, Pindborg J. Verrucous hyperplasia of the oral mucosa. Cancer 1980;46:1855–62.
6. Silverman S Jr, Gorsky M, Lozada F. Oral leukoplakia and malignant transformation: a long-term study of thirty patients. Cancer 1984;53:563–8.
7. Zakrzewska JM, Lopes V, Speight P, et al. Proliferative verrucous leukoplakia: a report of ten cases. Oral Surg Oral Med Oral Pathol Oral Radiol Endod 1996;82:396–401.
8. Cabay RJ, Morton TH, Epstein JB. Proliferative verrucous leukoplakia and its progression to oral carcinoma: report of three cases. J Oral Pathol Med 2007;36:315–8.
9. Bagan JV, Jiminez Y, Sanchis JM, et al. Proliferative verrucous leukoplakia: high incidence of gingival squamous cell carcinoma. J Oral Pathol Med 2003; 32:379–82.
10. Palefsky JM, Silverman S Jr, Abdel-Salaam M, et al. Association between proliferative verrucous leukoplakia and human papilloma virus 16. J Oral Pathol Med 1995;24:193–7.
11. Cabay RJ, Morton TH, Epstein JB. Proliferative verrucous leukoplakia and its progression to oral carcinoma: a review of the literature. J Oral Pathol Med 2007;36:255–61.
12. Campisi G, Giovanelli L, Ammatuna P, et al. Proliferative verrucous vs conventional leukoplakia: no significantly increased risk of HPV infection. Oral Oncol 2004;40:835–40.
13. Fettig A, Pogrel MA, Silverman S Jr, et al. Proliferative verrucous leukoplakia of the gingiva. Oral Surg Oral Med Oral Pathol Oral Radiol Endod 2000;90: 723–30.
14. Bagan JV, Jiminez Y, Murillo J, et al. Lack of association between proliferative verrucous leukoplakia

and human papilloma virus infection. J Oral Maxillo-fac Surg 2007;65:46–9.

15. Beltiol JC, Kignel S, Tristao W, et al. HPV 18 preva-lence in oral mucosa diagnosed with verrucous leu-koplakia: cytological and molecular analysis. J Clin Pathol 2012;65(8):769–70.

16. Kresty LA, Mallery SR, Knobloch TJ, et al. Frequent alterations of p16INK4a and p14ARF in oral prolifer-ative verrucous leukoplakia. Cancer Epidemiol Biomarkers Prev 2008;17:3179–87.

17. Olofsson J. Comment on DNA ploidy in proliferative verrucous leukoplakia. Oral Oncol 2007;43:621.

18. Gouvea AF, Vargas PA, Coletta RD, et al. Clinico-pathologic features and immune histochemical expression of p53, Ki-67, Mcm-2 and Mcm-5 in proliferative verrucous leukoplakia. J Oral Pathol 2010;39:447–52.

19. Murrah V, Batsakis JG. Proliferative verrucous leuko-plakia and verrucous hyperplasia. Ann Otol Rhinol Laryngol 1994;103:660–3.

20. Dougherty TJ, Henderson B. Historical perspective: Schwartz S, Winkelman JW, Lipson RL. In: Henderson BW, Dougherty TJ, editors. Photody-namic therapy. New York: Marcel Dekker Inc.; 1992. p. 1–15.

21. Doherty TJ, Gomer CJ, Henderson BW, et al. Photo-dynamic therapy. J Natl Cancer Inst 1998;90(12):889–905.

22. Lou PJ, Jones L, Hopper C. Clinical outcomes of photodynamic therapy for head-and-neck cancer. Technol Cancer Res Treat 2003;2(4):311–7.

23. Franco RA. Aminolevulinic acid 585 nm pulsed dye laser photodynamic treatment of laryngeal keratosis with atypia. Otolaryngol Head Neck Surg 2007;136(6):882–7.

24. Chen HM, Yu CH, Tu PC, et al. Successful treatment of oral verrucous hyperplasia and oral leukoplakia with topical 5-Aminolevulinic Acid-mediated photo-dynamic therapy. Lasers Surg Med 2005;37(2):114–22.

25. Chen HM, Chen CT, Yang H, et al. Successful treat-ment of an extensive verrucous carcinoma with topical 5-aminolevulinic acid-mediated photody-namic therapy. J Oral Pathol Med 2005;34(4):252–6.

26. Walvekar RR, Chaukar DA, Deshpande MS, et al. Verrucous Carcinoma of the oral cavity: a clinical and pathological study of 101 cases. Oral Oncol 2009;45(1):45–51.

27. Oliveira DT, de Moraes RV, Fiamengui F, et al. Oral verrucous carcinoma: a retrospective study in Sao Paulo region, Brazil. Clin Oral Investig 2006;10(3):205–9.

28. Femiano F, Gombos F, Scully C. Oral proliferative verrucous leukoplakia (PVL); open trial of surgery compared with combined therapy using surgery and methisoprinol in papillomavirus-related PVL. Int J Oral Maxillofac Surg 2001;30(4):318–22.

29. Nair MK, Sankaranarayanan R, Padmanabhan TK, et al. Oral verrucous carcinoma. Treatment with radiotherapy. Cancer 1988;61(3):458–61.

30. Koch BB, Trask DK, Hoffman HT, et al. National Survey of Head and Neck verrucous carcinoma: patterns of presentation, care and outcome. Cancer 2001;92(1):110–20.

31. Smucler R, Vlk M. Laser ablation vs "wait and see" in treatment of oral leukoplakia—10 years study. Lasers Surg Med 2012;44(Suppl 24):26 [abstract: #77].

32. Hong WK, Endicott J, Itri LM, et al. 13-Cis-retinoid acid in the treatment of oral leukoplakia. N Engl J Med 1986;315:1501–5.

33. Poveda-Roda R, Bagan JV, Jimenez-Soriano Y, et al. Retinoids and proliferative verrucous leukoplakia (PVL). A preliminary study. Med Oral Patol Oral Cir Bucal 2010;15(1):e3–9.

# Targeted Therapy in Head and Neck Cancer

Brent B. Ward, DDS, MD

## KEYWORDS

- Cancer • Nanotechnology • Chemotherapy • Radiation • Targeted therapy

## KEY POINTS

- Cervical lymph node metastasis is a major prognostic indicator in squamous cell carcinoma (SCC) of the head and neck.
- Sentinel node biopsy for SCC of the head and neck continues to be a controversial topic but studies have been undertaken that propose to validate the use of sentinel node biopsy for this purpose.
- Surgical margins positive for cancer are an indication for the addition of chemotherapy to postoperative radiation because of the significant increase in persistent disease.
- Transoral robotic surgery is an exciting advance in the care of patients, especially with early laryngopharyngeal and oropharyngeal cancer in which significant decreases in morbidity of treatment can be achieved.
- Surgeons should continue to seek the treatments that target tumors to the greatest extent possible such that efficacy is consistently maximized and the toxicity of the treatments is limited for improvements in both survival and quality of life.

## INTRODUCTION AND HISTORICAL PERSPECTIVE

The desire to target therapies to specific cancers is not new, although the use of the word has taken on greater prominence in recent years. The aim of targeting is to find the so-called silver bullet. The concept arises from folklore, in which a silver bullet was the only defense effective against many mystical foes. In modern terms, for cancer therapy, targeting refers to an effort to create therapies that specifically interact with diseased cells while leaving other tissues of the host untouched. In theory and in practice, targeted therapies either increase efficacy or decrease toxicity related to treatment. The most effective agents do both, but patients and doctors may be willing to tolerate increased toxicity for highly effective treatments or sacrifice efficacy for decreased toxicity. Such trade-offs must be carefully evaluated and tailored to individual patients and disease processes in an informed fashion.

A Medline search for targeted therapy or targeted drug delivery reveals the degree of interest and discovery in this field. Two articles from 1902 to 1978 are available, with the first mention attributed to the use of propranolol for essential hypertension by Lauro and colleagues[1] In the 1980s, 53 articles were published on targeted approaches, which expanded in the 1990s to 261. Since that time significant expansion of the use of this term has occurred with 1429 articles for targeted approaches from 2000 2006 and 8338 in the subsequent 6 years to 2012. Specific to cancer, this increase in enthusiasm for targeting is attributable to several factors, including expanding knowledge of the cancer process from a basic scientific perspective, increased throughput on patient-specific markers, advances in biomedical instrumentation, and technological advances that

Oral and Maxillofacial Surgery, Maxillofacial Oncologic and Reconstructive Surgery, University of Michigan, 1500 East Medical Center Drive, Ann Arbor, MI 48109-0018, USA
E-mail address: bward@umich.edu

Oral Maxillofacial Surg Clin N Am 25 (2013) 83–92
http://dx.doi.org/10.1016/j.coms.2012.11.006
1042-3699/13/$ – see front matter © 2013 Elsevier Inc. All rights reserved.

allow interaction with cancer cells in a more selective fashion.

Advances in understanding of the cellular and molecular changes leading to malignancy have assisted this revolution. In the 1950s, Foulds[2] conceptually elaborated the proposed mechanisms of tumor progression. These concepts were followed shortly by documentation of cytogenetic chromosomal changes in the 1960s. Molecular techniques evolved, as did cancer theory, resulting in the belief that tumorigenesis started from abnormalities in a single altered cell.[3] A multistep model with acquisition of various cellular abnormalities was eventually proposed.[4] Even without each step currently stipulated, global understanding of both the cancer cell and the importance of the surrounding milieu continues to expand. With these advances, there is recognition that, in addition to cancer transforming markers available for interaction with targeted approaches, nontransforming markers that are overexpressed for a variety of reasons may also be targeted to offer some selective advantages in cancer treatment. Considering the readership and task, this article focuses on targeted therapies for head and neck cancer in surgery, radiation, and chemotherapy as multimodality treatment of head and neck cancer.

## TARGETED SURGERY

In using the definition of targeting as defined earlier, advances of this type are not new. A well-known historical example introduces a discussion that focuses on current investigational strategies and future targeting strategies for head and neck cancer.

In the early 1900s, Crile[5,6] reported the first large series of patients undergoing radical en block neck dissections with a higher success rate than patients undergoing procedures that were less than en bloc. Prominent surgeons promoted radical neck dissection as the standard for treatment of this disease. It was not until the 1960s that modifications by Suárez, Bocca and others led to the modified radical neck dissection. Work by surgeons at MD Andersen Cancer Center first showed that treatment outcomes were similar in patients treated with radical neck dissections compared with selective neck dissections.[7] In recent years, the selectivity of neck dissections has become increasingly targeted, to a point at which some surgeons have proposed selective dissection of nodal basins in levels I to III for patients with N1/N2 disease.[8] The targeting in this clinical scenario leads to the removal of specific at-risk nodal basins. In this case, the targeting results in similar efficacy with decreased toxicity in the form of decreased surgical morbidity. Like many of the subsequent discussions, biomedical and instrumentation advances may contribute to future decreases in morbidity. Some examples include the emerging role of sentinel node biopsy and robotic surgery which was shown in a recent cadaver-based study of minimally invasive robotic-assisted neck dissection.[9] A review of neck dissection is an example of progress in targeting through decreased systemic toxicity from an ever-increasing desire to affect only the tumor in these treatments. This article considers sentinel node, advances in primary tumor margin control, and robotics as surgical targeting.

### Sentinel Node Biopsy

Cervical lymph node metastasis is a major prognostic indicator in squamous cell carcinoma (SCC) of the head and neck. In 1977, Cabanas introduced the concept of sentinel lymph node biopsy (SLNB), which in recent years has dramatically changed the treatment of some cancers. In the sentinel node approach, removal of major sets of lymph nodes is completed only in cases of advanced disease or when the sentinel lymph node, harvested in a minimally invasive fashion, is found to be positive for cancer.

The sentinel node refers to the first or a small set of initial nodes draining a cancer within the body. This node is assumed to be the gatekeeper (sentinel), such that its tumor status indicates the probability of other, more distant, nodal involvement. If cancer has not spread to the sentinel node, then the likelihood of other nodal involvement is presumed to be low. The reliability of this technique has been proved in melanoma, including melanoma of the head and neck, as well as breast cancers, and remains under study in several other cancers (including SCC of the head and neck).

Sentinel node mapping generally is performed using 2 modalities. First, preoperative planar lymphoscintigraphy uses a low-activity radionuclide injected at the site of the tumor, followed by serial scintigraphic imaging until the sentinel node is identified, which is followed by intraoperative γ probe/Geiger meter detection to identify radioactive, or hot, nodes. Second, the injection of a visual blue dye at the site of cancer just before operation, which leads to blue dye visualization in the draining lymph nodes at the time of neck exploration. Nodes are generally reported as hot, blue, or hot and blue, indicating the presence or absence of radioactivity and blue dye uptake (Fig. 1). The sentinel node(s) harvested can then be carefully examined not only histopathologically

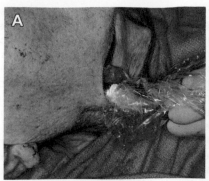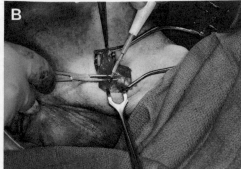

**Fig. 1.** (*A*) The use of a γ probe with a minimal neck incision for identification of a sentinel lymph node with (*B*) subsequent removal. (*Courtesy of* R. Bryan Bell.)

but with immunohistochemistry and molecular examination for micrometastasis and conventional metastasis of cancer.

Sentinel node biopsy for SCC of the head and neck continues to be a controversial topic but several studies have been undertaken to validate the use of sentinel node biopsy for this purpose. In 2010, a prospective multi-institutional trial for SLNB was reported involving 25 institutions over a 3-year period with the accrual of 140 patients with T1/T2 primaries and clinically N0 necks. The patient population included 95 cancers of the tongue, 26 of the floor of mouth, and 19 other oral cancers. Exclusion criteria included lesions less than 6 mm and lesions with minimal invasion (although a criterion for minimal invasion was not defined in the report). In the protocol, all patients underwent sentinel node biopsy followed by a formal neck dissection for the purpose of defining the negative-predictive value (NPV) of SLNB. Of the 106 SLNBs that were negative on hematoxylin and eosin staining, 100 patients were without additional nodal disease (NPV 94%). NPV was increased to 96% with additional sectioning and immunohistochemistry. For patients found to have positive nodal disease in the neck on formal dissection, the true-positive rate or sensitivity overall of the sentinel node was 90.2%, indicating that, in approximately 10% of cases, the sentinel node was negative but the neck overall was positive. The breakdown of these falsely negative nodes revealed a sensitivity of 85% for T2 and 100% for T1 lesions. The sentinel node performed better on tongue lesions than lesions of the floor of the mouth. Surgeons designated prospectively as experienced also had a false-negative rate of 0. Overall, the study provided much to consider given the generally accepted cutoff of 20% risk for performing formal neck dissection. The lack of clarity regarding the minimally invasive lesion is important because many surgeons approach depth of invasion as an indication for neck dissection in T1 lesions. The results reported for experienced surgeons and T1 lesions are without false-negatives but questions remain regarding appropriate application as attempts are made to generalize the study to individual patients.[10]

Melkane and colleagues[11] recently reported a 10-year experience with oral SCC, having accumulated a cohort of 166 patients between 2000 and 2010 with a mean follow-up period of 36 months. Sentinel node involvement was highest in tongue cancers versus floor of mouth (34% vs 13%, $P = .003$), advancing tumor stage (18% positive for T1 vs 40% for T2, $P = .002$), median depth of invasion (6.5 mm for positive vs 4 mm for negative, $P = .028$) and lymphovascular involvement ($P = .002$). The false-negative rate of standard frozen section examination was 42%, with 14 of the patients harboring only micrometastases.

Overall, the current literature suggests that the predictive value of a negative SLNB is 90% to 100%, that serial step sectioning with immunohistochemistry is critical to achieve this outcome, and that SLNB may assist in upstaging patients who might not generally undergo formal neck dissection (including the ability to identify abnormal drainage patterns that may alter the surgical plan). Concerns remain about the false-negative rate potentially related to the possibility of skip metastasis, the learning curve associated with this technique, and a lack of level I evidence to support its use.[12] Technological advances in this area include studies of novel tracers and improving the throughput of results that would obviate 2 separate surgical interventions in patients found to have a positive sentinel node.

## Margin Control

Clean surgical margins remain the goal of cancer resection surgery. Surgical margins positive for cancer are an indication for the addition of chemotherapy to postoperative radiation because of the significant increase in persistent disease. In addition, some evidence suggests that margins with mild to moderate dysplasia likewise increase the risk of recurrence.[13] Much has been written and reported about what constitutes a clean margin; that discussion is beyond the scope of this article. Regardless, attempts to fine-tune the ability to define the margin constitute targeting; this is an example of targeting in which additional toxicity is generally accepted in the form of larger resections with the goal of increased efficacy in long-term tumor control.

Toluidine blue staining has been investigated as a technique for diagnosis of oral SCCs and epithelial dysplasia for many years with variable reported outcomes. In addition, toluidine blue has been reported as a tool for obtaining clean surgical margins, and recently as a replacement for frozen section analysis in locations where frozen section is not feasible. Junaid and colleagues[14] reported a comparative analysis of toluidine blue and frozen section in 56 consecutive patients with 280 tumor margins. Eleven margins stained positive for toluidine blue, and, of these margins, 3 were positive on frozen or final pathology. There were no false-negatives, indicating that toluidine blue may overpredict the needed resection but did not underpredict in any of the cases in the study. In this application, toluidine blue had a sensitivity of 100% with a specificity of 97% owing to the small number of false-positives in which toluidine blue overpredicted the needed margin. The routine use of toluidine blue for surgical margins is not standard but is an indication of the possibilities that exist in the quest for better margin control.

Kurita and colleagues[15] reported the use of tissue staining with indigo carmine and Congo red with assessment of the deep surgical margin in comparison with hematoxylin and eosin staining as the gold standard. The extent of carcinoma could be accurately visualized in 80% of the specimens, with no significant difference between the tumor-stained margin and the histopathologic margin. Staining in this way may decrease the randomness in choosing locations for frozen section analysis and thereby decrease the risk of false-negative results.

Fluorescence visualization has been examined as an adjunct to visual examination in the operating room to determine surgical margins. In their protocol, Poh and colleagues[16] first examined 20 oral cavity lesions planned for resection under white light marking the anticipated surgical margin, which was followed by autofluorescence examination and an additional marking of margins.

Following excision around both margins, the fluorescent visualization loss (FVL)–guided region was examined for histologic and genetic changes. In 19 of the 20 specimens, FVL changes extended beyond the clinically visible lesions. Thirty-two of the 36 biopsies in these areas revealed changes from mild/moderate dysplasia to SCC. Molecular analysis of biopsies with low-grade or no dysplasia revealed loss of heterozygosity markers 3p and/or 9p, which have been associated with tumor recurrence. Although this study only provides proof of principle, a well-designed, randomized, multicenter, double-blind, controlled surgical trial evaluating the use of the addition of fluorescence visualization in surgical margin control is underway. The study anticipates the recruitment of 160 cases of severe dysplasia or carcinoma in situ and 240 invasive cancers. The study end point is local recurrence following resection with patients followed for up to 5 years. The results of this study will give a high level of evidence either in favor or against the use of this technique to more adequately address surgical margins.

Genetic analysis applications have also been studied as a form of margin control. For example, Heah and colleagues[17] studied immunohistochemistry and fluorescent in situ hybridization of the tumor suppressor TP53 gene in the margins of 26 oral SCCs, showing that 96% of excisions contained genetic alterations at the excision margins. Other genetic analyses have included chromosomal changes with multiplex ligation-dependent probe amplification, loss of heterozygosity with microsatellite polymerase chain reaction, and DNA index alterations using DNA image analysis.[18] Shaw and colleagues investigated quantitative methylation at resection margins and lymph nodes using pyrosequencing methylation assays (PMA) of CpG islands within the gene promoter of p16 and CYGB genes. PMA upgraded 13 of the 20 surgical margins, 6 of which eventually recurred. Although the study population and adjuvant treatments made firm conclusions difficult, this provides another potential avenue for molecular marker margin control.

## Transoral Robotic Surgery

The introduction of robotic-assisted surgery has transformed minimally invasive surgery in a variety of surgical disciplines. Several advantages to this approach have been proposed in head and neck SCC. These advantages include the decreased need for access surgery with large incisions and the ability to surgically treat diseases in a minimal surgical fashion that were previously amenable to treatment only with chemotherapy and radiation therapy organ preservation protocols because of associated surgical morbidity.

Robotic surgery was first introduced in the mid 1980s. Multiple advances since that time have led to the current da Vinci Surgical System (Intuitive Systems, Sunnyvale CA), which is the most common robotic system in use today. Robotic surgery uses optics and instrumentation with varying degrees of rotation such that access can be achieved to the base of tongue and entire pharyngeal region as well as access to portions of the larynx. A single-institution report on the use of transoral robotic surgery (TORS) in 54 patients with laryngopharyngeal SCC with 11.8 months' follow-up was retrospectively evaluated. There were no major intraoperative complications and no aborting of any procedure because of an inability to remove the cancer. A 7% positive margin rate was noted. All patients tolerated an oral diet on the day of surgery and no airway compromise was noted. The investigators concluded that TORS spared patients radiation therapy or combined chemotherapy and radiation in 50% of stage I/II tumors. In addition, chemotherapy was spared in 34% of stage III/IV tumors. These results indicate a significant decrease in overall morbidity for patients treated for their disease with TORS.[19]

A multicenter study evaluating the feasibility, safety, and surgical margins of TORS reviewed early results from 3 institutions that had undertaken prospective clinical trials using TORS. Of 177 total patients, 78% had oropharynx tumors and 26% tumors of the larynx. Nineteen percent of the tumors were malignant, with 95% of these being SCC. Most were early lesions (T1 32.7%, T2 48.4%, T3 13.7%, and T4 5.2%). The average follow-up was almost 1 year. The rate of positive surgical margins was 4.3%. There were 34 serious adverse events requiring hospitalization but none of these were deemed to be directly related to the use of TORS.[20]

Additional detailed information is available in an article specifically dedicated to TORS by Eric and colleagues in this issue. In summary, TORS is an important advance in the care of patients, especially those with early laryngopharyngeal and oropharyngeal cancer in which significant decreases in morbidity of treatment can be achieved. At present, long-term functional data and data for oncologic safety are lacking, but what has accumulated to date is encouraging.

## TARGETED RADIATION

The complex anatomy and multitude of adjacent critical structures creates complexities for radiation therapy for the head and neck. For example, the spinal cord, brainstem, and optic system are barriers in terms of dose. In addition, quality-of-life issues arise when high doses of radiation lead to changes in taste, hearing, speech, and oral/pharyngeal function related to swallowing. Although several strategies exist to target radiation delivered specifically to the tumor bed while protecting outlying structures, this article discusses only intensity-modulated radiotherapy (IMRT) as an example of advances in targeted radiation therapy. IMRT is an example of targeting in which there is the possibility of increased efficacy through higher radiation doses to tumor beds. In addition, similar efficacy with decreasing toxicity because of decreased radiation to adjacent structures has been extensively documented.

IMRT is a high-precision radiotherapy developed in recent years that uses computer-controlled linear accelerators to modulate the intensity of each beam of radiation (**Fig. 2**). In addition, it uses multiple ports of entry that conform the radiation three-dimensionally to the tumor bed. The combination of these approaches leads to maximal radiation in the specific desired location while minimizing radiation to surrounding tissues. This targeted approach to radiation allows higher doses to be directed to the tumor with significant decreased morbidity to surrounding structures. Treatment planning of these regimens uses images in isolation or combination from computed tomography, magnetic resonance imaging, and positron emission tomography to create three-dimensional plans for radiation delivery by noting the tumor bed as a desired site for high-intensity radiation and marking sites with desired sparing so that computer plans can be generated. Given the preciseness of the plan, patients are often fitted with a radiation mask that immobilizes the sites of interest during treatment, because even slight movements create deviation from the computer-generated plan and thereby deliver radiation to an undesired location.

A recent systematic review by O'Sullivan and colleagues[21] highlights some of the advantages of IMRT compared with standard external beam radiation therapy, specifically as it relates to decreased toxicity. The review included 14 studies in total, with 3 randomized controlled trials providing the highest levels of evidence. The reviewed data led to 4 specific recommendations, 3 of which suggested a benefit of IMRT compared with standard external beam radiation therapy. IMRT was recommended to decrease xerostomia, blindness, and osteoradionecrosis (ORN) as side effects of treatment. There was not strong

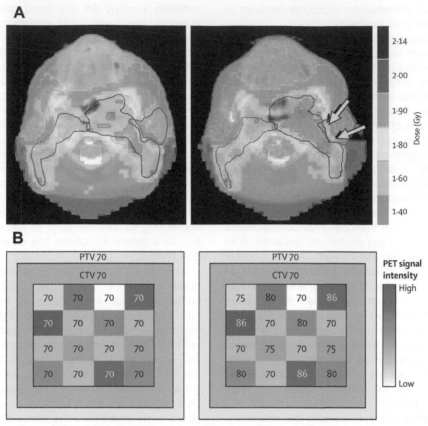

**Fig. 2.** Conformal planned and delivered dose (*A*) and example of dose painting technology (*B*), which are available with IMRT technology. Arrows indicate the overdose of the left parotid gland compared with the planned dose. CTV, clinical target volume; PTV, planning target volume. (*From* Grégoire V, Jeraj R, Lee JA, et al. Radiotherapy for head and neck tumours in 2012 and beyond: conformal, tailored, and adaptive? Lancet Oncol 2012;13(7):e292–300; with permission.)

evidence in the studies reviewed for treatment benefit, and therefore the guidelines concluded that IMRT is, at worst, not inferior to standard radiation therapy. Taken as a whole, IMRT offers clinically relevant and statistically significant reductions in adverse event rates with associated increases in quality of life. The author's experience mirrors these findings, particularly as it relates to xerostomia and a decreased, but not zero, rate of ORN. These data and experience give rise questions for which additional data are not available to provide definitive answers. As an example, what is the success rate of implants in native mandible and free flaps for patients receiving IMRT versus standard external beam radiation? At our institution we have experienced greater numbers of implant failures in patients who have sought their radiation from centers that do not have expertise in IMRT. In the limited number of cases in which implant failure ultimately led to ORN and loss of bone segments, failure occurred in patients who did not receive IMRT. In light of the data and

experience, all patients at our primary institution receiving adjunctive radiation therapy in addition to surgery receive IMRT. We offer strong encouragement to patients who require radiation treatment elsewhere to pursue only locations where IMRT can be delivered and where expertise in IMRT specifically for the head and neck is available.

## TARGETED CHEMOTHERAPY

Advances in surgery and radiation presently provide, and have great additional potential for, augmented targeting through combination with targeted chemotherapeutic strategies. Until recently, chemotherapy was limited to cytotoxic agents specifically designed against cell replication, thus taking advantage of constant tumor growth. These drugs were generally nonspecific; for example, common chemotherapeutic agents like cisplatin (inducing DNA damage), fluorouracil (focused on DNA replication), and taxanes (disrupting the process of cell division). Advances in basic and translational research have brought increased understanding of both cell surface and cell signaling changes in cancer, as well as the local environmental requirements (tumor microenvironment), which have produced several possibilities for a more targeted chemotherapeutic approach. In addition, advances in drug delivery strategies that capitalize on interacting specifically with tumor cells hold great promise. Although the development of these technologies is slow, they likely hold the greatest promise for disease control in the future. For simplicity, this article focuses on proof-of-principle examples in a vast field of ever-increasing potential applications.

## Epidermal Growth Factor Receptor

Epidermal growth factor receptor (EGFR) was discovered in the 1950s and is a member of the HER/erbB family of receptor tyrosine kinases. On binding one of its ligands (eg, epidermal growth factor receptor [EGFR] or transforming growth factor [TGF]-$\alpha$), the EGFR forms homodimers, or heterodimers with the other family members, leading to the activation of the intrinsic receptor tyrosine kinase enzyme activity. Mutations or high expression levels of EGFR have been identified in many cancer types, including lung, colon, breast, and head and neck. In these diseased tissues, the autophosphorylation of EGFR leads to the activation of downstream signaling pathways and nuclear expression of multiple molecules that eventually lead to cell proliferation, angiogenesis, tumor invasion, and metastasis.[22,23] More than 90% of head and neck cancers show overexpression of EGFR, making this abnormality very common and an excellent candidate for targeting.[24]

Several EGFR inhibitors have been tested in the clinic, with additional preclinical candidates under study. The landmark phase III trial by Bonner and colleagues[25] using cetuximab (Erbitux; ImClone Systems, Bristol-Myers Squibb and Merck, New York, NY), a monoclonal antibody to EGFR, was the first to offer evidence of increased efficacy for radiation therapy when combined with a targeted chemotherapeutic. Patients with locally advanced disease were randomized to receive radiation therapy in conjunction with cetuximab versus radiation therapy alone as control. Both progression-free and overall survival were improved with the addition of the targeted chemotherapeutic. The success of the trial by Bonner and colleagues[25] has prompted several additional studies using cetuximab with radiation or cetuximab in addition to chemoradiation with fluorouracil and platinum-based chemotherapies in which the addition of cetuximab has likewise showed a clinical benefit.[26,27] However, the studies related to cetuximab have been controversial. For example, some patients in the initial trial received different radiotherapy regimens and the trial had no comparison with standard chemoradiation, which has also been showed to have survival benefit in some patients. In addition, the emergence of human papillomavirus–related cancers and their potential effect on the results of studies for which this was an unaccounted variable have the potential to invalidate any positive results. However, cetuximab remains the flagship of targeted chemotherapy in head and neck SCC and an excellent example of the length of time it takes to achieve clinical use, with more than 50 years from discovery to phase III clinical validation.

The success of cetuximab has led to several other attempts to interact with EGFR at the extracellular domain, including the monoclonal antibodies panitumumab (Vectibix, Amgen, Thousand Oaks, CA; approved in colorectal cancer and under evaluation in head and neck SCC), zalutumumab (HUMax-EGFR, Genmab, Copenhagen, Denmark), and nimotuzumab (BIOMAb EGFR, Biocon, India; Theracim, YM biosciences, Cuba; Theraloc, Oncosciences, Europe; CIMaher, Cuba), which are currently under study. In addition, the use of small-molecule inhibitors that interact with the intracellular activity of EGFR have been studied in phase II and III trials. Gefitinib (Iressa, AstraZeneca Pharmaceuticals, London, UK) is directed against the intracellular domain of EGFR. A phase II trial using gefitinib showed some benefit to patients with recurrent disease but this result has not been replicated in phase III endeavors. Several similar agents are in phases I to III, with none validated for routine clinical use at the present time.

## Vascular Endothelial Growth Factor

Vascular endothelial growth factor (VEGF) is an example of targeting using the increased need for angiogenesis of tumors compared with normal tissue. There are several VEGFs, each binding to a tyrosine kinase receptor for activity. Increased VEGF expression has been correlated with a decrease in overall and progression-free survival as well as lymph node metastasis.[28,29] Similar to EGFR, attempts have been made to target both the extracellular receptor through monoclonal antibodies, and intracellular pathways through small-molecule inhibitors. Bevacizumab (Avastin, Genetech/Roche, San Francisco, CA) is approved by the US Food and Drug Administration for colorectal and lung cancer and has been studied in patients with head and neck SCC. Several phase I and II trials have been reported with promising results in efficacy and toxicity. For example, in a phase II Radiation Therapy Oncology Group (RTOG) trial, patients who had the addition of bevacizumab to the regimen of chemoradiation had fewer distant metastases than historical controls.[30] In the small-molecule inhibitor realm, cediranib (AZD2171, Recentin, AstraZeneca, London, UK) has been given to patients with non–small cell lung cancer with some demonstrated effect, but studies specific to head and neck SCC have been disappointing.

## Mammalian Target of Rapamycin

Mammalian target of rapamycin (mTOR) is an example of potential targeting that benefits from a wide range of basic and preclinical translational supportive science leading to its current early clinical phase. mTOR is a highly conserved seronine/threonine kinase that plays a role in the PI3K/AKT signaling pathway involved in cell growth, proliferation, and survival. Aberrant regulation of the mTOR pathway has been shown in head and neck SCC as well as several other tumors.[31] Rapamycin is a natural macrolide antibiotic and immunosuppressant with demonstrated antitumor effects. Years of research and development have resulted in the development of 3 rapamycin analogues with enhanced pharmacologic properties: temsirolimus, everolimus, and deforolimus. Most trials to date have been based on patients with renal cell carcinoma, in whom promising results have been obtained, leading to enthusiasm for translation to head and neck SCC. At present, several phase II trials evaluating mTOR inhibitors in patients with head and neck SCC are currently recruiting patients.[32]

## Nanotargeted Chemotherapy

Nanotechnology offers the unique opportunity of developing personalized therapeutics based on targeting and treating specific receptors and abnormalities of a patient's tumor. As predicted by the National Cancer Institute, it is likely that nanotechnology will enhance all current aspects of cancer prevention, detection, and treatment. Nanotargeted chemotherapy to head and neck SCC is one representative area of research in an ever-growing field of basic science seeking better targeted approaches in chemotherapy. Scientific discovery in tumor pathways, receptors, and microenvironment, as well as the creation and optimization of pharmaceutical

approaches, all contribute to this field. The author's personal experience represents a vast array of research endeavors likely to change the landscape of cancer treatment in the decades to come.

Dendrimers or dendritic polymers are uniform spherical nanostructures ranging from 10 to 200 Å in diameter. Dendrimers possess several advantages compared with other drug delivery vehicles in their small size, globular shape, multiple ligand valence capacity, flexibility, and stability. Dendrimers have served as a platform to which the attachment of several types of biologic materials has been validated. Examples of functional attachments have included iron oxide for targeted imaging, phiphiluxG1D2 apoptosis sensor for monitoring, drugs including methotrexate and taxol chemotherapeutics, and folic acid, RGD peptides, EGF, and antibody fragments for targeting. The structure, connection, and numbers of targeting molecules are pivotal to the ultimate function of these drug delivery devices. Dendrimers for cancer have been validated using folate for targeting and methotrexate for chemotherapy (**Fig. 3**). In a cell line that overexpresses the high-affinity folate receptor, in vitro and in vivo xenograft mouse tumor models for targeted methotrexate chemotherapy showed a 10-fold to 50-fold increase in efficacy with a significant decrease in systemic toxicity compared with free drug.[33,34] This example therefore both increases efficacy and decreases toxicity, which is the ultimate goal for optimal targeting. Translating these findings to preclinical models in head and neck SCC has required the ability to ascertain folate receptor activity in several cell lines followed by animal model validation of therapeutic effect. Screening a large number of cell lines in head and neck SCC showed a scalable array of expression that, when put into animal models, showed direct correlation with tumor control (ie, no expression having no benefit from targeting, moderate expression having moderate effect, and high expression having high efficacy of drug). Preclinical validation was achieved using folate receptor–targeted chemotherapy with methotrexate in a mouse xenograft model in which both increased efficacy and decreased toxicity were confirmed compared with free drug. This report represented the first translation of nanotargeted chemotherapy with dendrimer to a clinically relevant preclinical tumor model.[35]

Expanding on this technology, creation of a multitude of devices specific to both the desired target and the desired chemotherapeutic may be possible. For example, a tumor high in EGFR and with high sensitivity to taxol could be treated with

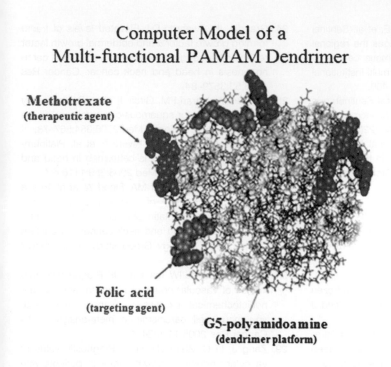

## Computer Model of a Multi-functional PAMAM Dendrimer

**Methotrexate** (therapeutic agent)

**Folic acid** (targeting agent)

**G5-polyamidoamine** (dendrimer platform)

**Fig. 3.** Computer model of nanodevice for targeted chemotherapy with folic acid targeting and methotrexate chemotherapy. (*From* Ward BB, Dunham T, Majoros IJ, et al. Targeted dendrimer chemotherapy in an animal model for head and neck squamous cell carcinoma. J Oral Maxillofac Surg 2011;69(9):2452–59; with permission.)

dendrimer bound to EGF and taxol. In other patients with either different targets or sensitivity to alternative agents, the device could be specifically created to treat their particular tumors. Further devolvement in dendrimer chemotherapeutics and tumor screening would combine to enable a tumorcentric regimen for any given patient. In addition, the ability to have dendrimers with imaging-sensing and apoptosis-sensing capabilities raises the possibility of a single therapeutic that not only treats tumor but documents its presence and ultimate eradication.

## SUMMARY AND FUTURE DIRECTIONS

Targeting of treatments to head and neck SCC is continually advancing. For the purposes of this article, targeting is discussed under the headings of surgical, radiation, and chemotherapeutic targeting. It is likely that no single technique will ultimately resolve the issues for all patients with head and neck cancer, but that a contribution from each will create the synergism needed for advances in the care of these patients. Surgeons should continue to seek the treatments that target tumor to the maximum extent possible, such that efficacy is consistently maximized and the toxicity of treatments is limited for both survival and quality-of-life improvements. Robust scientific discovery will undoubtedly yield the greatest benefit to patients with cancer.

## REFERENCES

1. Lauro R, Platania A, Liberatore C, et al. Biochemical profile of essential arterial hypertension. Indications for a targeted therapy: experience with propranolol. Clin Ter 1978;85(1):19–25 [in Italian].
2. Foulds L. Tumor progression. Cancer Res 1957;17:355–6.
3. Nowell PC. The clonal evolution of tumor cell populations. Science 1976;194:23–8.
4. Vogelstein B, Kinzler KW. The multistep nature of cancer. Trends Genet 1993;9:138–41.
5. Crile GW. Excision of cancer of the head and neck with special reference to the plan of dissection based on one hundred and thirty-two operations. JAMA 1906;47:1780–6.
6. Crile GW. On the surgical treatment of cancer of the head and neck. With a summary of one hundred and twenty-one operations performed upon one hundred and five patients. Trans South Surg Gynecol Assoc 1905;18:108–27.
7. Jesse R, Ballantyne AJ, Larson D. Radical or modified neck dissection: a therapeutic dilemma. Am J Surg 1978;136:516–9.
8. Battoo AJ, Hedne N, Ahmad SZ, et al. Selective neck dissection is effective in N1/N2 nodal stage oral cavity squamous cell carcinoma. J Oral Maxillofac Surg 2012. [Epub ahead of print].
9. Blanco RG, Ha PK, Califano JA, et al. Robotic-assisted neck dissection through a pre- and post-auricular hairline incision: preclinical study. J Laparoendosc Adv Surg Tech A 2012;22(8):791–6.

10. Civantos FJ, Zitsch RP, Schuller DE, et al. Sentinel lymph node biopsy accurately stages the regional lymph nodes for T1-T2 oral squamous cell carcinomas: results of a prospective multi-institutional trial. J Clin Oncol 2010;28(8):1395–400.

11. Melkane AE, Mamelle G, Wycisk G, et al. Sentinel node biopsy in early oral squamous cell carcinomas: a 10-year experience. Laryngoscope 2012;122(8):1782–8.

12. Civantos FJ, Stoeckli SJ, Takes RP, et al. What is the role of sentinel lymph node biopsy in the management of oral cancer in 2010? Eur Arch Otorhinolaryngol 2010;267(6):839–44.

13. Weijers M, Snow GB, Bezemer PD, et al. The clinical relevance of epithelial dysplasia in the surgical margins of tongue and floor of mouth squamous cell carcinoma: an analysis of 37 patients. J Oral Pathol Med 2002;31(1):11–5.

14. Junaid M, Choudhary MM, Sobani ZA, et al. A comparative analysis of toluidine blue with frozen section in oral squamous cell carcinoma. World J Surg Oncol 2012;10:57.

15. Kurita H, Sakai H, Kamata T, et al. Accuracy of intraoperative tissue staining in delineating deep surgical margins in oral carcinoma surgery. Oral Oncol 2008;44(10):935–40.

16. Poh CF, Zhang L, Anderson DW, et al. Fluorescence visualization detection of field alterations in tumor margins of oral cancer patients. Clin Cancer Res 2006;12(22):6716–22.

17. Heah KG, Hassan MI, Huat SC. p53 Expression as a marker of microinvasion in oral squamous cell carcinoma. Asian Pac J Cancer Prev 2011;12(4):1017–22.

18. Bremmer JF, Braakhuis BJ, Brink A, et al. Comparative evaluation of genetic assays to identify oral precancerous fields. J Oral Pathol Med 2008;37(10):599–606.

19. Hurtuk A, Agrawal A, Old M, et al. Outcomes of transoral robotic surgery: a preliminary clinical experience. Otolaryngol Head Neck Surg 2011;145(2):248–53.

20. Weinstein GS, O'Malley BW Jr, Magnuson JS, et al. Transoral robotic surgery: a multicenter study to assess feasibility, safety, and surgical margins. Laryngoscope 2012;122(8):1701–7.

21. O'Sullivan B, Rumble RB, Warde P, Members of the IMRT Indications Expert Panel. Intensity-modulated radiotherapy in the treatment of head and neck cancer. Clin Oncol 2012;24:474–87.

22. Lurje G, Lenz HJ. EGFR signaling and drug discovery. Oncology 2009;77:400–10.

23. Yarden Y, Sliwkowski MX. Untangling the ErbB signaling network. Nat Rev Mol Cell Biol 2001;2:127–37.

24. Grandis JR, Tweardy DJ. Elevated levels of transforming growth factor α and epidermal growth factor receptor messenger RNA are early markers of carcinogenesis in head and neck cancer. Cancer Res 1993;53:3579–84.

25. Bonner JA, Harari PM, Giralt J, et al. Radiotherapy plus cetuximab for squamous-cell carcinoma of the head and neck. N Engl J Med 2006;354:567–78.

26. Vermorken JB, Mesia R, Rivera F, et al. Platinum-based chemotherapy plus cetuximab in head and neck cancer. N Engl J Med 2008;359:1116–27.

27. Burtness B, Goldwasser MA, Flood W, et al. Phase III randomized trial of cisplatin plus placebo compared with cisplatin plus cetuximab in metastatic/recurrent head and neck cancer: an Eastern Cooperative Oncology Group study. J Clin Oncol 2005;23:8646–54.

28. Kyzas PA, Cunha IW, Ioannidis JP. Prognostic significance of vascular endothelial growth factor immunohistochemical expression in head and neck squamous cell carcinoma: a meta-analysis. Clin Cancer Res 2005;11:1434–40.

29. Zang J, Li C, Zhao LN, et al. Prognostic value of vascular endothelial growth factor in patients with head and neck cancer: a meta-analysis. Head Neck 2012. http://dx.doi.org/10.1002/hed.23156.

30. Lee N, Zhang Q, Garden A, et al. Phase II study of chemoradiation plus bevacizumab (BV) for locally/regionally advanced nasopharyngeal carcinoma (NPC): preliminary clinical results of RTOG 0615. ASCO annual meeting. J Clin Oncol 2011;29:5516.

31. Molinolo AA, Hewitt SM, Amornphimoltham P, et al. Dissecting the Akt/mammalian target of rapamycin signaling network: emerging results from head and neck cancer tissue array initiative. Clin Cancer Res 2007;17:4964–73.

32. Nguyen SA, Walker D, Gillespie MB, et al. mTOR inhibitors and its role in the treatment of head and neck squamous cell carcinoma. Curr Treat Options Oncol 2012;13(1):71–81.

33. Quintana A, Raczka E, Piehler L, et al. Design and function of a dendrimer-based therapeutic nanodevice targeted to tumor cells through the folate receptor. Pharm Res 2002;19:1310–6.

34. Kukowska–Latallo J, Candido KA, Cao Z, et al. Nanoparticle targeting of anticancer drug improves therapeutic response in animal model of human epithelial cancer. Cancer Res 2005;65:5317–24.

35. Ward BB, Dunham T, Majoros IJ, et al. Targeted dendrimer chemotherapy in an animal model for head and neck squamous cell carcinoma. J Oral Maxillofac Surg 2011;69(9):2452–9.

# Oral Lichen Planus

Justin Au, DMD, MD*, Dhaval Patel, DDS,
John H. Campbell, DDS, MS

## KEYWORDS

- Lichen planus • Oral • Autoimmune disease • Reticular • Erosive

## KEY POINTS

- Lichen planus is an immunologically mediated mucocutaneous disease, affecting 0.1% to 4% of the general population.
- Several reports suggest an association of hepatitis C virus and human papilloma virus with oral lichen planus.
- Oral lichen planus predominately affects females, with most patients aged between 30 and 70 years.
- Common treatment options include systemic and topical corticosteroids, topical retinoids, cyclosporine, tacrolimus, and pimecrolimus.
- The potential malignant transformation of lichen planus remains highly controversial; periodic observation of these lesions for dysplastic changes remains prudent.

## INTRODUCTION

Lichen planus is an immunologically mediated mucocutaneous disease. A complex series of immunologic events is purported to cause the initiation and perpetuation of the condition. It is a common disease, affecting 0.1% to 4.0% of the general population. Patients often have concomitant cutaneous and oral lesions (**Fig. 1**).[1,2] Oral lesions may be chronic in nature, remitting and relapsing with varying degrees of morbidity; they range from asymptomatic to debilitating pain.

Clinically and histologically similar entities, including lichenoid drug reaction (**Fig. 2**), lichenoid mucositis (**Fig. 3**), and lichenoid dermatitis, can make the diagnosis of lichen planus challenging. These lesions are associated with the administration of a drug or direct contact with a metal and often, but not always, resolve when the offending agent is removed. Antibiotics, antihypertensives, gold, diuretics, antimalarials, and nonsteroidal antiinflammatory drugs may precipitate these conditions.[3] Oral lichenoid reactions in chronic graft-versus-host disease are also well recognized.[4,5] It is not possible to distinguish such lesions from oral lichen planus (OLP) clinically or histologically; there is, however, a significantly higher frequency of CD25+ cells in the epithelium and the connective tissue of OLP than in chronic graft-versus-host disease. This variance in frequency indicates differences in regulatory mechanisms of the immunologic response in the two conditions.[6] Genetic involvement in OLP is yet to be determined.[7,8]

Several reports suggest an association of hepatitis C virus and human papilloma virus with OLP.[9,10] In Spain and Japan, there is a reported incidence of coinfection of 20% and 62%, respectively, with HCV; but this has not been shown in the American population.[11–13]

## CLASSIFICATION

The classification of lichen planus is based on clinical presentation and is divided into 3 main

The authors have nothing to disclose.
Department of Oral and Maxillofacial Surgery, University at Buffalo, 3435 Main Street, 112 Squire Hall, Buffalo, NY 14215, USA
* Corresponding author.
E-mail address: justinau@buffalo.edu

oralmaxsurgery.theclinics.com

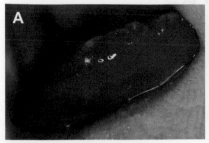
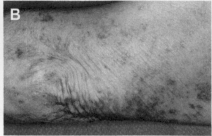

**Fig. 1.** (*A*) Superficial ulcer of erosive lichen planus on the lateral border of the tongue. Note atrophic appearance of the tongue. (*B*) Skin lesions on the extensor surface of the arm and forearm in the same patient as (*A*).

forms: reticular, erosive, and atrophic (or erythematous) lesions. Many other descriptors have also been used, including bullous, plaquelike, and papular. There is often overlap between types, with a combination of reticular, erosive, and erythematous lesions.

## CLINICAL FEATURES

OLP predominately affects females, with most patients aged between 30 and 70 years.[11] It is a rare occurrence in children; but in men, lesions often develop at an earlier age. The presentation is varied in clinical appearance, with most lesions being bilateral and located on the buccal mucosa. Lesions can appear, however, on the tongue, in the vestibule, and on the gingivae. Isolated gingival lichen planus may be seen in up to 8.6% of patients.[12,13]

Malignant transformation of lichen planus is highly controversial.[14–16] The term *premalignant* implies eventual malignant transformation, but lichen planus may better be described as having "malignant potential."[16] There has been a reported incidence of 0.4% to 1.5% malignant transformation to squamous cell carcinoma in patients with lichen planus.[17] The World Health Organization's (WHO) criteria describe lichen planus as a condition predisposed to malignant transformation.[18]

Others have suggested that another entity, known as lichenoid dysplasia, is responsible for the conversion to malignancy. These lesions are dysplastic leukoplakias with a secondary lichenoid infiltrate but are often misdiagnosed as lichen planus.[15] It is also purported that patients with erosive lichen planus are more susceptible to known carcinogenic agents because of the lack of an epithelial barrier. Regardless, most investigators advocate periodic observation for dysplastic changes.

### Reticular Lichen Planus

Reticular lichen planus is the most common type and is often found incidentally. Lesions are asymptomatic and located on the buccal mucosa, tongue, gingivae, or in the vestibule.[2] The lesions present as white, slightly raised plaques or papules with interlacing white lines described as Wickham striae on an erythematous background.

### Erosive Lichen Planus

Erosive lichen planus appears atrophic, with areas of ulceration, erythema, and keratotic white striae. There can be pseudomembranes, and in the gingival region it often appears similar to desquamative gingivitis. There is a range of symptoms, from a mild burning sensation to debilitating pain. Lesions can interfere with speech, chewing, and

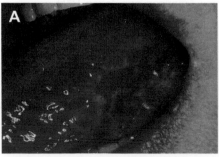
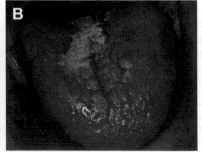

**Fig. 2.** (*A*) Superficial ulceration mimicking lichen planus in a patient taking nonsteroidal antiinflammatory medication. (*B*) Lichenoid lesions in a patient using nonsteroidal antiinflammatory medication. The lesions resolved after stopping the drug.

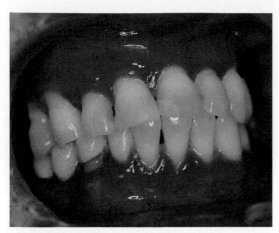

**Fig. 3.** Lichenoid stomatitis of gingivae, thought to be allergic in nature.

swallowing. These lesions can be mixed with reticular lesions, which are not seen in other vesiculoerosive diseases, such as pemphigus, pemphigoid, and linear immunoglobulin A (IgA) disease.[19]

## Erythematous, Atrophic Lichen Planus

This form of lichen planus presents as a red, diffuse lesion with mucosal atrophy.

## Plaquelike Lichen Planus

Solitary, slightly raised, or flat white lesions appear similar to leukoplakia; a common oral location is on the tongue (**Fig. 4**).

## Bullous Form

This rare form of OLP exhibits bullae that rupture, progressing to erosive lichen planus.

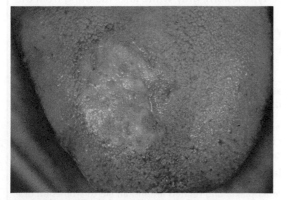

**Fig. 4.** Plaquelike lichen planus on the dorsum of the tongue.

## CAUSE

Although the exact cause is not known, the literature supports an inflammatory immune cause for OLP.[20–23] An antigen-specific cell-mediated immune response, autoimmune response, and humoral immunity have been previously described as mediating factors along with nonspecific mechanisms.[24–27] The antigen-specific cell-mediated immune response involves CD8+ T cells triggering keratinocyte apoptosis via the caspase cascade pathways.[28–30] Keratinocyte apoptosis further triggers alteration in the basement membrane, causing nonspecific T-cell migration into the epithelium from the subepithelial layer. Altered basement membrane, matrix metalloproteinase (MMP), chemokines,[25] and mast cells are part of the nonspecific mechanisms proposed in the development of OLP.[27,31] T cells produce and secrete regulated on activation, normal T-Cell expressed and secreted (RANTES), a chemokine that enhances mast cell destruction, leading to the release of tumor necrosis factor–$\alpha$ and chymase. This loop is a positive feedback loop that further stimulates RANTES production.[32] RANTES is also involved in the recruitment of lymphocytes, monocytes, natural killer cells, eosinophils, basophils,[32] and mast cells. Chymase activates MMP-9 that, in turn, causes basement membrane disruption.[33] Keratinocyte-derived transforming growth factor–$\beta$1 mediates a weak immune response and upregulation of heat shock proteins and of circulating humoral antibodies against desmogleins 1 and 3 in OLP.[25,34] The response may be autoimmune in nature[35] or may be associated with exogenous antigens.[26,36,37]

## HISTOLOGY

Dubreuil was the first to describe the histopathology of OLP in 1906; in 1972, Shklar reported the classic histologic features of overlying keratinization, a dense bandlike layer of lymphocytic infiltrate within the underlying connective tissue, and liquefaction degeneration of the basal cell layer.[38] Current literature supports common findings of dense, well-defined infiltrate of lymphocytes in the superficial dermis, orthokeratotic hyperkeratosis, parakeratosis, acanthosis, epithelial atrophy, basal cell degeneration[39] and saw-tooth rete pegs.[20,25] Homogeneous eosinophilic globules, known as colloid bodies (Civatte, hyaline, or cytoid), are found at the degenerating basal keratinocyte layer.[20,25] The dense bandlike lymphocytic infiltration of the superficial stroma, basal epithelial cell liquefactive degeneration, and colloid bodies are considered the key features of OLP.[24] The presence of plasma cells and B cells is uncommon. Hemidesmosomes, filaments, and fibrils forming the epithelial anchoring system at the basal layer show disturbances.[40] These disturbances produce deterioration of the epithelial-connective tissue junction leading to the formation of clefts called Max-Joseph spaces.[25] Fibrin and fibrinogen in a linear pattern at the basal membrane layer is a common finding on direct immunofluorescence.[24] Colloid bodies stain positively with IgM, C3, and C4. These immunofluorescence findings are highly suggestive of, although not diagnostic for, OLP when associated with other histologic features.[24,41] The final diagnosis of OLP is concluded by clinical and histopathologic presentation.[15,26]

The WHO published the clinical and histopathologic diagnostic criteria of OLP (**Box 1**) in 1978.[42] However, they have recently been assessed for their validity given the current controversy with the premalignant nature of OLP.[41] Some investigators have made recommendations (**Box 2**) to improve the diagnostic assessment of OLP based on clinical and histologic features.[15,41]

## TREATMENT AND PROGNOSIS

The management of lichen planus can be difficult. Cochrane evidence is weak for all interventional modalities.[43] There is no cure, and most therapeutic modalities aim for symptomatic relief (**Fig. 5**). This disease is a chronic disease, with periods of remission and relapse. The reticular form of lichen planus, when asymptomatic, does not require treatment. Common treatment options include systemic and topical corticosteroids, topical retinoids, cyclosporine, tacrolimus, and pimecrolimus.

Eisen[12] found that exacerbation of the disease was precipitated by stress, foods, dental procedures, systemic illness, and poor oral hygiene. Oral lesions improved or resolved when the exacerbating factor was removed.[12] Avoidance of irritating factors and improvement of periodontal health can aid in the management of these lesions.

Systemic corticosteroids are an important form of treatment of diffuse erosive lichen planus or in patients who are refractory to topical steroids. There are, however, many side effects, even with short-term use. These side effects include hyperglycemia, diabetes, osteoporosis, cataracts, depression, hypertension, hypothyroidism, and amenorrhea.[44] Systemic steroids can be used alone or in combination with topical corticosteroids, but they have not been found to be more effective than topical triamcinolone acetonide alone.[44–46] In fact, topical triamcinolone acetonide alone has been shown to be an equally or more effective treatment in patients with erosive lichen planus.[47] There are many effective formulations, including Orabase, lozenges, pastes, or mouthwash.[48,49] Other topical corticosteroids (fluocinonide, betamethasone, clobetasol gel) have also been used with success. The side-effect profiles of topical corticosteroids are less severe than systemic corticosteroids but can include opportunistic candidiasis; mucosal atrophy; and, in cases of high-potency topical steroids, adrenal suppression.[50,51]

Betamethasone as an oral mini-pulse therapy (2 consecutive days per week) has been shown

---

**Box 1**
**WHO diagnostic criteria (1978) for diagnosis of OLP**

*Clinical Criteria*

Presence of white papule, reticular, annular, or plaque-type lesions, gray-white lines radiating from the papules

Presence of a lacelike network of slightly raised gray-white lines (reticular pattern)

Presence of atrophic lesions with or without erosion may also have bullae

*Histopathologic Criteria*

Presence of a thickened orthokeratinized or parakeratinized layer in sites that are normally keratinized; layer may be very thin if site is normally nonkeratinized

Presence of Civatte bodies in basal layer, epithelium, and superficial part of the connective tissue

Presence of a well-defined, bandlike zone of cellular infiltration that is confined to the superficial part of the connective tissue, consisting mainly of lymphocytes

Signs of liquefaction degeneration in the basal cell layer

*From* Kramer IR, Lucas RB, Pindborg JJ, et al. Definition of leukoplakia and related lesions: an aid to studies on oral precancer. Oral Surg Oral Med Oral Pathol 1978;46(4):518–39; with permission.

---

**Box 2**
**Proposal for a set of modified WHO diagnostic criteria of OLP and OLL**

*Clinical Criteria*

There is the presence of bilateral, more or less symmetric lesions.

There is the presence of a lacelike network of slightly raised gray-white lines (reticular pattern).

Erosive, atrophic, bullous, and plaque-type lesions are accepted only as a subtype in the presence of reticular lesions elsewhere in the oral mucosa.

In all other lesions that resemble OLP but do not complete the aforementioned criteria, the term *clinically compatible with* should be used.

*Histopathologic Criteria*

There is the presence of a well-defined bandlike zone of cellular infiltration that is confined to the superficial part of the connective tissue, consisting mainly of lymphocytes.

There are signs of liquefaction degeneration in the basal cell layer.

There is an absence of epithelial dysplasia.

When the histopathologic features are less obvious, the term *histopathologically compatible with* should be used.

*Final Diagnosis OLP or OLL*

To achieve a final diagnosis, clinical as well as histopathologic criteria should be included.

OLP: A diagnosis of OLP requires fulfillment of both clinical and histopathologic criteria.

OLL: The term OLL will be used under the following conditions:

1. Clinically typical of OLP but histopathologically only compatible with OLP
2. Histopathologically typical of OLP but clinically only compatible with OLP
3. Clinically compatible with OLP and histopathologically compatible with OLP

*Abbreviation:* OLL, oral lichenoid lesions.
*From* van der Meij EH, van der Waal I. Lack of clinicopathologic correlation in the diagnosis of oral lichen planus based on the presently available diagnostic criteria and suggestions for modifications. J Oral Pathol Med 2003;32(9):507–12; with permission.

---

to be as effective as topical triamcinolone acetonide paste. This therapy has a lower side-effect profile than conventional systemic corticosteroids, and its use for exacerbations or as monotherapy has been described as effective.[52]

Intralesional injections of hydrocortisone, dexamethasone, triamcinolone acetonide, and methylprednisolone have also been used with short-term success.[53] These injections are, however, often painful and can inadvertently cause mucosal atrophy.[24]

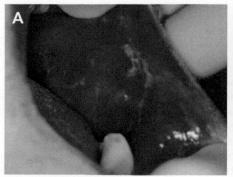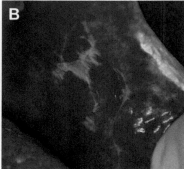

**Fig. 5.** (*A*) Painful and ulcerated lesion of lichen planus before treatment. (*B*) Same patient as in (*A*), after treatment with chlorhexidine. Pain, ulcer, and erythema have resolved.

Patients with lichen planus can have superimposed candidiasis infections or can be secondarily infected with candidiasis from corticosteroid therapy.[54] Treatment of *Candida* can help prevent exacerbations and can convert the erosive form to the reticular form.[55] Further, corticosteroid-related candida infections can be treated with concomitant topical miconazole gel therapy.[56]

Retinoids in topical or systemic forms have been used in the treatment of OLP. They are best used as an adjuvant therapy and have a significant recurrence rate after discontinuation of the drug.[57]

Cyclosporin is an immunosuppressant that affects T-cell cytokine production. Its use as a topical or mouth rinse in treatment of OLP has been reported with mixed results.[58,59] Disadvantages include poor patient compliance because of taste, a burning sensation, and expense.

Pimecrolimus is an immunosuppressant agent in the ascomycin class of macrolactams. It inhibits T-cell activation and proliferation by acting on the calcineurin pathway.[60] Gorouhi and colleagues[60] found topical pimecrolimus cream four times a day to be as effective as triamcinolone acetonide paste. Tacrolimus is in the same drug class as pimecrolimus. Topical tacrolimus has a smaller molecular mass than cyclosporine and can better penetrate the epidermal barrier to exert its effect. It has been shown to have an equivalent or better initial therapeutic response than triamcinolone acetonide for treating erosive lichen planus but also shows greater relapse when therapy is discontinued.[61–65]

Other treatments that have been reported include antibiotics, antimalarials, azathioprine, dapsone, glycyrrhizin, interferon, levamisole, mesalazine, and phenytoin.[17] Many of these drugs, however, are also known to induce lichenoid reactions themselves. Recently, Mansourian and colleagues[66] has shown aloe vera to be an effective substitute for triamcinolone acetonide as a topical treatment. The antioxidant properties of aloe vera have antiinflammatory, analgesic, and antiproliferative effects.[66]

## SUMMARY

OLP is a very common immunologically mediated disease. It has varied clinical presentations and can appear on the buccal mucosa, tongue, gingivae, or in the vestibule. The common forms are reticular, erosive, and erythematous patterns. Management is aimed at symptomatic relief and includes systemic and topical corticosteroids, retinoids, tacrolimus, and pimecrolimus. The potential malignant transformation of lichen planus remains highly controversial. Periodic observation of these lesions for dysplastic changes remains prudent.

## REFERENCES

1. Altman J, Perry HO. The variations and course of lichen planus. Arch Dermatol 1961;84:179–91.
2. DeRossi SS, Ciarrocca KN. Lichen planus, lichenoid drug reactions, and lichenoid mucositis. Dent Clin North Am 2005;49(1):77–89, viii.
3. Giunta JL. Oral lichenoid reactions versus lichen planus. J Mass Dent Soc 2001;50(2):22–5.
4. Nakamura S, Hiroki A, Shinohara M, et al. Oral involvement in chronic graft-versus-host disease after allogeneic bone marrow transplantation. Oral Surg Oral Med Oral Pathol Oral Radiol Endod 1996;82(5):556–63.
5. Eckardt A, Starke O, Stadler M, et al. Severe oral chronic graft-versus-host disease following allogeneic bone marrow transplantation: highly effective treatment with topical tacrolimus. Oral Oncol 2004;40(8):811–4.
6. Hasseus B, Jontell M, Brune M, et al. Langerhans cells and T cells in oral graft versus host disease and oral lichen planus. Scand J Immunol 2001;54(5):516–24.
7. Carrozzo M, Francia Di Celle P, Gandolfo S, et al. Increased frequency of HLA-DR6 allele in Italian patients with hepatitis C virus-associated oral lichen planus. Br J Dermatol 2001;144(4):803–8.
8. Carrozzo M, Uboldi de Capei M, Dametto E, et al. Tumor necrosis factor-alpha and interferon-gamma polymorphisms contribute to susceptibility to oral lichen planus. J Invest Dermatol 2004;122(1):87–94.
9. Mattila R, Rautava J, Syrjanen S. Human papillomavirus in oral atrophic lichen planus lesions. Oral Oncol 2012;48(10):980–4.
10. Lodi G, Giuliani M, Majorana A, et al. Lichen planus and hepatitis C virus: a multicentre study of patients with oral lesions and a systematic review. Br J Dermatol 2004;151(6):1172–81.
11. Jaafari-Ashkavandi Z, Mardani M, Pardis S, et al. Oral mucocutaneous diseases: clinicopathologic analysis and malignant transformation. J Craniofac Surg 2011;22(3):949–51.
12. Eisen D. The clinical features, malignant potential, and systemic associations of oral lichen planus: a study of 723 patients. J Am Acad Dermatol 2002;46(2):207–14.
13. Scully C, el-Kom M. Lichen planus: review and update on pathogenesis. J Oral Pathol 1985;14(6):431–58.
14. van der Meij EH, Schepman KP, Smeele LE, et al. A review of the recent literature regarding malignant transformation of oral lichen planus. Oral Surg Oral Med Oral Pathol Oral Radiol Endod 1999;88(3):307–10.

15. Eisenberg E. Oral lichen planus: a benign lesion. J Oral Maxillofac Surg 2000;58(11):1278–85.

16. Silverman S Jr. Oral lichen planus: a potentially premalignant lesion. J Oral Maxillofac Surg 2000; 58(11):1286–8.

17. Lodi G, Scully C, Carrozzo M, et al. Current controversies in oral lichen planus: report of an international consensus meeting. Part 2. Clinical management and malignant transformation. Oral Surg Oral Med Oral Pathol Oral Radiol Endod 2005;100(2):164–78.

18. Pindborg JJ, Wahi PN. Histological typing of cancer and precancer of the oral mucosa. In: International histological classification of tumours. 2nd edition. Berlin: Springer; 1997. p. 87.

19. Rhodus NL, Myers S, Kaimal S. Diagnosis and management of oral lichen planus. Northwest Dent 2003;82(2):17–9, 22–5.

20. Farhi D, Dupin N. Pathophysiology, etiologic factors, and clinical management of oral lichen planus, part I: facts and controversies. Clin Dermatol 2010;28(1): 100–8.

21. Kawamura E, Nakamura S, Sasaki M, et al. Accumulation of oligoclonal T cells in the infiltrating lymphocytes in oral lichen planus. J Oral Pathol Med 2003; 32(5):282–9.

22. Yamamoto T, Nakane T, Osaki T. The mechanism of mononuclear cell infiltration in oral lichen planus: the role of cytokines released from keratinocytes. J Clin Immunol 2000;20(4):294–305.

23. Iijima W, Ohtani H, Nakayama T, et al. Infiltrating CD8+ T cells in oral lichen planus predominantly express CCR5 and CXCR3 and carry respective chemokine ligands RANTES/CCL5 and IP-10/ CXCL10 in their cytolytic granules: a potential self-recruiting mechanism. Am J Pathol 2003;163(1): 261–8.

24. Scully C, Beyli M, Ferreiro MC, et al. Update on oral lichen planus: etiopathogenesis and management. Crit Rev Oral Biol Med 1998;9(1):86–122.

25. Sugerman PB, Savage NW, Walsh LJ, et al. The pathogenesis of oral lichen planus. Crit Rev Oral Biol Med 2002;13(4):350–65.

26. Ismail SB, Kumar SK, Zain RB. Oral lichen planus and lichenoid reactions: etiopathogenesis, diagnosis, management and malignant transformation. J Oral Sci 2007;49(2):89–106.

27. Lodi G, Scully C, Carrozzo M, et al. Current controversies in oral lichen planus: report of an international consensus meeting. Part 1. Viral infections and etiopathogenesis. Oral Surg Oral Med Oral Pathol Oral Radiol Endod 2005;100(1):40–51.

28. Jungell P, Konttinen YT, Nortamo P, et al. Immunoelectron microscopic study of distribution of T cell subsets in oral lichen planus. Scand J Dent Res 1989;97(4):361–7.

29. Sugerman PB, Savage NW, Zhou X, et al. Oral lichen planus. Clin Dermatol 2000;18(5):533–9.

30. Mattila R, Syrjanen S. Caspase cascade pathways in apoptosis of oral lichen planus. Oral Surg Oral Med Oral Pathol Oral Radiol Endod 2010;110(5): 618–23.

31. Chainani-Wu N, Silverman S Jr, Lozada-Nur F, et al. Oral lichen planus: patient profile, disease progression and treatment responses. J Am Dent Assoc 2001;132(7):901–9.

32. Zhao ZZ, Sugerman PB, Zhou XJ, et al. Mast cell degranulation and the role of T cell RANTES in oral lichen planus. Oral Dis 2001;7(4):246–51.

33. Zhou XJ, Sugerman PB, Savage NW, et al. Matrix metalloproteinases and their inhibitors in oral lichen planus. J Cutan Pathol 2001;28(2):72–82.

34. Lukac J, Brozović S, Vucicević-Boras V, et al. Serum autoantibodies to desmogleins 1 and 3 in patients with oral lichen planus. Croat Med J 2006;47(1): 53–8.

35. Sugerman PB, Satterwhite K, Bigby M. Autocytotoxic T-cell clones in lichen planus. Br J Dermatol 2000;142(3):449–56.

36. Muller S. Oral manifestations of dermatologic disease: a focus on lichenoid lesions. Head Neck Pathol 2011;5(1):36–40.

37. Schlosser BJ. Lichen planus and lichenoid reactions of the oral mucosa. Dermatol Ther 2010; 23(3):251–67.

38. Shklar G. Lichen planus as an oral ulcerative disease. Oral Surg Oral Med Oral Pathol 1972; 33(3):376–88.

39. Jungell P, Konttinen YT, Malmstrom M. Basement membrane changes in oral lichen planus. Proc Finn Dent Soc 1989;85(2):119–24.

40. Haapalainen T, Oksala O, Kallioinen M, et al. Destruction of the epithelial anchoring system in lichen planus. J Invest Dermatol 1995;105(1): 100–3.

41. van der Meij EH, van der Waal I. Lack of clinicopathologic correlation in the diagnosis of oral lichen planus based on the presently available diagnostic criteria and suggestions for modifications. J Oral Pathol Med 2003;32(9):507–12.

42. Kramer IR, Lucas RB, Pindborg JJ, et al. Definition of leukoplakia and related lesions: an aid to studies on oral precancer. Oral Surg Oral Med Oral Pathol 1978;46(4):518–39.

43. Cheng S, Kirtschig G, Cooper S, et al. Interventions for erosive lichen planus affecting mucosal sites. Cochrane Database Syst Rev 2012;(2):CD008092.

44. Carbone M, Goss E, Carrozzo M, et al. Systemic and topical corticosteroid treatment of oral lichen planus: a comparative study with long-term follow-up. J Oral Pathol Med 2003;32(6):323–9.

45. Vincent SD, Fotos PG, Baker KA, et al. Oral lichen planus: the clinical, historical, and therapeutic features of 100 cases. Oral Surg Oral Med Oral Pathol 1990;70(2):165–71.

Printed and bound by CPI Group (UK) Ltd, Croydon, CR0 4YY

03/10/2024

01040347-0005